It's Never Too Late to Be Healthy

It's Never Too Late to Be Healthy

Reaching Peak Health in Middle Age

Kevin Brady

TESTIMONIALS

"As a fellow plant-strong triathlete, it's great how Kevin has represented Canada the last 5 years at the World Triathlon Championships fuelled by a plant-based diet and a golden attitude. It's never too late to benefit from the lessons Kevin shares in this terrific book!" –Rip Esselstyn, triathlete, health activist and author of *The Engine 2 Diet*, *The Engine 2 Seven-Day Rescue Diet* and *Plant-Strong*

"I have known Kevin for over 22 years, and I can say he looks in better shape and healthier today than he did when I first met him. His book provides actionable steps to help readers live a healthier and happier life." –Dan Sullivan, Co-Founder and President of Strategic Coach, author of more than 30 books, including his recent book *Who Not How: The Formula to Achieve Bigger Goals Through Accelerating Teamwork*

"This is one of those books with information that is ready to use. A handy book to have in your home and business." –T. Colin Campbell, PhD, Jacob Gould Schurman Professor Emeritus of Nutritional Biochemistry at Cornell University and co-author of *The China Study*

"We all want to be healthy but having a guide on a difficult journey is the wisest plan. *It's Never Too Late to be Healthy* provides the path of experience to lead you to a successful upgrade to your total health. Start this today, see your vitality blossom." –Joel Kahn, MD, FACC, holistic cardiologist and author of *The Plant-Based Solution*

"With encouragement and instruction on how to get restorative sleep, reduce stress, incorporate gentle but effective exercise, as well as how to find your community in which to contribute and enjoy life-affirming fellowship, *It's Never Too Late To Be Healthy* delivers hope and motivation to its readers. This small but powerful book will be a welcome roadmap for all who are on their life's journey to better health and I heartily recommend it." –Dr. Michael Klaper, director of Moving Medicine Forward Initiative, physician, consultant, educator and author

"The pursuit of good health requires a decision and commitment on the part of the individual, but the support of a community dedicated to peoples' well-being makes the journey easier and goals more achievable. The YMCA has known this throughout its 165-plus-year history, and we are delighted to see Kevin's story expressing this truth so clearly." –Medhat Mahdy, President and CEO of the YMCA of Greater Toronto

It's Never Too Late to Be Healthy: Reaching Peak Health in Middle Age

Copyright © 2021 by Advica Health

Paperback ISBN 978-1-7774809-0-5
Ebook ISBN 978-1-7774809-1-2

Disclaimer
This book is a general guide only and should never be a substitute for the skill, knowledge, and experience of a qualified medical professional dealing with the facts, circumstances and symptoms of a particular case. The nutritional, medical, and health information presented in this book is based on the research, training and professional experience of the author, and is true and complete to the best of his knowledge. However, this book is only intended as an informative guide for those wishing to know more about health, nutrition, and wellbeing; it is not intended to replace or countermand the advice given by the reader's personal physician and/or personal qualified health care provider. Because each person and situation is unique, the author and the publisher urge the reader to check with a qualified health-care professional before using any procedure where there is a question as to its appropriateness. A physician should be consulted before beginning any exercise program. The author and the publisher are not responsible for any adverse effects or consequences resulting from the use of the information in this book and assumes no responsibility for any liability, loss or risk, personal or otherwise. It is the responsibility of the reader to consult a physician or other qualified health-care professional regarding his or her personal care.

Design & Production: Alexandra Battey, Julie Inc. Author Consulting & Marketing
Consulting Editor: Fina Scroppo
Editorial Assistant: Vanessa Silano
Copyeditor: Suzanne Robertson-Moutis
Cover Design & Illustrations: Lauren Brady
Recipe Development Assistant: Barb Brady and Sheena Rollan
(See References section for excerpted recipes)

All inquiries should be addressed to:

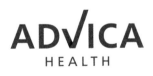

Advica Health
2115 S Service Rd W, Oakville, ON L6L 5W2
+1 888-598-7655
www.advicahealth.com
k.brady@advicahealth.com

If you're interested in bulk purchases of It's Never Too Late to Be Healthy, we offer an aggressive discount schedule. Please call us at the number listed.

Printed in Canada on 100% post-consumer recycled paper

Dedication

To my parents, Joanie and Howie. You showed me love, courage and confidence throughout my life.

To my amazing wife, Barb. I have been in love with you since the first day we met. I love your positive disposition and your ongoing support.

To our children, Tim, Matt and Lauren. You have always inspired me to be the best I can be, and I'm continually motivated and learning from you.

To all of my family, the "rock" in my life. I love you all and thank you for being "you." You are truly the most amazing gift one could ever ask for.

I'd also like to dedicate this book to the YMCA, which has a special place in my heart. I began attending YMCA camps at the age of 8, and today I'm proud to say I'm still a member along with my entire family. Our involvement in their programs has had a tremendous impact on our lives, helping to build our mind, body, and spirit throughout the years. In gratitude, I'm donating proceeds of the sale of EVERY book to the YMCA's children and youth programs.

XO

Contents

Foreword   1
Introduction   5
How to Use This Book   12

Part 1: The Early Years   **15**
    Don't Drink and Die   15
    Getting In Tune with Wellness   28

Part 2: The Wheels of Health   **37**
    The Keys to Your Health Transformation   37
    Wheel 1: Eating Well   41
    Wheel 2: Exercise   58
    Wheel 3: Sleep   66
    Wheel 4: Mindfulness   75

Part 3: The Health Action Plan   **87**
    Building Communities   87
      Step 1: Health Navigation   88
      Step 2: Reflect Back   98
      Step 3: Become a Health Citizen   105

Part 4: Resources, Routines & Recipes   **117**
    Build Your Resources   117
    Follow Routines   119

    Recipes   **125**
      Power Breakfast   126
      Vegan Mains   128
      Soups, Salads & Sides   152
      Desserts   168

The Wheels of Health Daily Log   172
Kevin's Top Picks   175
References   177

FOREWORD
By Rich Roll

I am the guy who could have used this book a dozen years ago, when I found myself 50 pounds overweight and struggling up the stairs, panting for breath. Although I had been a competitive swimmer in my youth, I found myself heading toward middle age as a sedentary lawyer on the verge of a heart attack.

At 39, I had been clean and sober for eight years, but I thought nothing of polishing off a plate of cheeseburgers followed by a pack of nicotine gum. I felt like I deserved it. After all, I wasn't drinking or doing drugs, and I worked hard. I deserved junk food. I had just cleaned up a second helping of ice cream and cake, trudged up the stairs to my daughter's room, and felt my heart pounding with effort. That was the night I had an epiphany.

Something big had to change. Otherwise, the risk that I wouldn't live long enough to see my daughter or stepsons grow up was real, and my wife, Julie, would be a widow. Much like Kevin had his game-changing moment, I had mine, and it led me down a much different path than I had expected.

The next day, I started to change my life in small ways, leading me to who I am today: an author, vegan, ultramarathoner, and podcaster. None of it would have been possible without simply making a start and putting one metaphoric foot in front of the other. That's why you need to read this book. You will learn that embracing a healthier lifestyle is not as daunting as it might seem. Like the power of compound interest that multiplies your finances over time, small daily actions can have a hugely positive effect on your long-term health and well-being.

Health is wealth. In our modern culture, especially as men, we're trained to chase the dollar and climb the corporate ladder. The true understanding of what it is to live a life of wellness doesn't come into focus until we suffer a crisis or calamity. This is about the only thing that precipitates a shuffling of priorities and gets us off our Habitrails. This applies particularly to men of a certain generation who have never spent much time thinking of their health and well-being in this context. But times are finally changing, albeit slowly. It's incumbent on all of us to take stock of what our day-to-day lives and habits look like.

Women are often faced with dual duties at home and work, which squeeze both time and energy from their day. Cooking whole foods, preparing meals ahead of time, exercising, and building a routine may seem impossible to the childless entrepreneur, single working mom, or married CEO. And women labor under a layer of guilt—they are usually more involved in the health care of family members and so understand perhaps better than men of a certain generation what is at stake.

We have a crisis of time management in our culture that few executives, of any gender, are immune to. It is far too easy to put off dealing with your own health and wellness when you have employees, shareholders, stakeholders, families, and loved ones who rely on you. It's too easy to say to yourself, "I just need to get through the next project or deadline, and then I promise to deal with my health."

The truth is, you *don't* have to put off self-care, nor should you. The time is *now*. This book is designed to help you make small daily changes to your lifestyle, diet, and outlook, which will take the pain out of that inevitable procrastination. These tiny shifts will help you move the needle in the right direction, and they won't take up any more time than you're currently spending—or not—to meet your health and wellness goals. Okay, they might take a little more time than doing nothing. But trust me, the eventual cost of doing nothing will be far greater and more time consuming than implementing small, daily changes now.

A lot of people feel like it's indulgent to take care of themselves when they have so much responsibility on their shoulders. That's fine, if you want to continue to live in the land of short-term gains, but it's not a great long-term strategy. Ultimately, you have to prioritize your self-care. Only then can you be better and more effective at supporting the people who depend on you and love you.

I know many of us feel like dealing with our health is a sign of weakness. It makes us feel vulnerable, so we push it away to some barely warm back burner. But it's not an understatement to say that we have as much need to think about and to care for our health as fit people do! In fact, it's imperative we do. So, rather than shoving that pain in your left kidney aside for the third week in a row, let your Type A personality get expressed in other, more positive ways.

I always tell people that mastering your plate, meaning what you eat every day, is the first place to start. However, you may have a pristine diet but aren't sleeping at night and end up being a jerk to your family. In that case, mindfulness and meditation may be the best place to start.

I have a couple of mantras I use. One of my favorites is *Don't let perfection be the enemy of progress*. People decide to lose 20 pounds or run a 10k, but when they're confronted with a setback, they faceplant into a pint of Häagen-Dazs, losing sight of the long-term goal. The key to not losing focus along the way is to change the way you look at these slipups and see them as positive experiences rather than failures. Look yourself in the mirror and say, "Whoops," then put your pants on one leg at a time.

Also, just begin. Lots of us suffer from analysis paralysis. Don't spend the next five years examining all the choices. This will just result in you being stuck in a circle of confusion and not making any. Instead, just begin, and follow the crumbs on the trail laid out in front of you. Especially when it comes to fitness. All those mental gymnastics are a barrier to actually *doing* the thing. As human beings, we are very good at overcomplicating things.

Another mantra I like is *Mood follows action*. This is when we say, "I don't feel like doing this or that today. I'll feel better tomorrow." The best way to shift that mindset is to take the action you're resisting. By doing so, you inhabit the mood that you were waiting for from the beginning. Set aside the ruminations of the thinking mind and just get moving. Shut down the familiar patterns in your head and push yourself beyond your comfort zone. Remember, the pattern may be there, but it doesn't mean you have to engage with it. It only carries the weight in your life you decide to give it.

I've known Kevin Brady for several years now. We met right after my book *Finding Ultra: Rejecting Middle Age, Becoming One of the World's Fittest Men, and Discovering Myself* was published. Kevin reached out to me, and we struck up an email friendship. I liked him immediately. Kevin is one of the most enthusiastic and engaging people I've met. He believed in me and brought me to Toronto for a speaking engagement about my book, putting together an amazing experience and hosting me and my family while we were there. We've stayed in touch ever since.

Kevin embraces these mindset shifts and more. This book is a little gem of 'what ifs.' What if you just took a walk every day at lunch? What if you started eating greens for lunch? What if you went to bed an hour earlier? What if you cut yourself some slack and just moved forward with reasonable health goals?

Kevin offers the hows to all these questions and more. Take this journey with Kevin—you'll be glad you did.

INTRODUCTION

I'm surrounded by men and women who work long hours every week, get little sleep, eat out all the time, and spend what little downtime they have in hotels in between attending conferences and seeing long-distance clients. Living fast-track lives and consuming fast food is bad enough, but combining these lifestyle choices with stress and no sleep can lead to health crises. Just the other day, I met with an exhausted business owner. I happened to mention he looked tired, and he said, "I woke up at 2 in the morning." He laughed and added, "I never got back to sleep."

It's not a laughing matter.

The four leading chronic causes of death in North America in descending order are heart disease, cancer, chronic lower respiratory disease, and diabetes. All four are exacerbated by obesity, which is now a worldwide epidemic. Couple all that with the fact that, with all our handheld devices, we don't even need a couch anymore to be couch potatoes; it's clear we have a major health crisis on our hands, and it's ballooning out of control.

We all want to be healthy. We all know we need to eat better and exercise more. The diet industry rakes in billions of dollars a year and fitness businesses alone score another $72 billion. Those amounts don't include classes and apps, as well other products that millions of walkers, runners, and cyclists out there use trying to stay fit while working out.

And yet, the unhealthy results just keep trending upward at an unnerving incline. Nearly every day, I see people who are struggling with their health, and they don't really know what to do. They are locked in a very common pattern of guilt, diet restriction, guilt, gym memberships, guilt, snacking, guilt, and eating the way they used to while their commitment to their workouts evaporates. They've tried different exercises and different diets, with often limited or temporary success, and they don't know how to get healthy and feel better overall. They've even attempted to get a better quality or quantity of sleep with some kind of aid but they're unsuccessful. It's a dangerous cycle they can't seem to break.

Too little sleep leads to poor performance in the short term and catastrophic health implications in the long term. Dementia is just one of a host of diseases affiliated with consistently getting too little sleep. People I know and communicate with are worn out, frustrated, and know they are not living a healthy lifestyle.

On the other hand, I also know people—friends, parents, business people, and professionals—who are trying to take care of themselves by eating right and exercising more. In my work as founder and CEO of Advica Health, a health and wellness company that connects people to a global network of premium health-care providers for their health issues, I often hear about the efforts individuals are making.

In fact, just this week one of our clients, who owns several automotive dealerships, said, "Kev, I need your help. I need to find a way to get healthy and fit again."

People like this client might look like they are in fairly good shape, with maybe "just a few pounds to lose." They get to the gym two, three, four days a week. Perhaps more. Perhaps they even run 10ks, half- or full marathons.

But they are not as healthy as they could be. In fact, they may not be healthy at all.

I WAS ONE OF THOSE PEOPLE

I ran marathons, I went to the gym, and I thought my diet was pretty good. In my 30s, I seemed to be on a sustainable path to a long life and good health.

I wasn't.

I had to figure out how to improve my health. Even after a near-death experience, I didn't fully change my ways until years later, when I was once again faced with my mortality. I learned never to take my health for granted, and I learned that quickly. It took a lot longer to figure out what to do about diet and exercise. Over time, my process and results began to open doors I never imagined, and I found myself in a position to influence the health of those around me in ever-increasing circles of the community. What started off as concerted efforts after a wake-up call has turned into a calling itself. I am fitter and in better overall health now at 58 than I was at 48, 38, or even 28.

I want to help others see the kind of success I've had. But it's hard to capture the imagination of people who already believe they are on the right path. Part of the problem is the revolving door of diets: Atkins, paleo, keto, high-fat, low-fat, no-carb, no-sugar—not to mention the oddball ones like the water diet, the avocado diet, the fruit diet. The rules of these diets are often inflexible, and the gurus who endorse them require complete adherence or the dieter will face failure. In other words, it's all or nothing. And even then, the diets don't work.

Then more guilt sets in. When I'm at dinner with colleagues, they often joke about what's on my plate or explain why they're eating all fried foods, or red meat, or having that second slice of cheesecake. I don't judge, though, because they're already trying to justify it themselves. They've put themselves in the food dog-house, and guilt is a terrible motivator. They know, on some level, that what they're eating probably isn't going to lead them down a healthy path. Paradoxically, they all know they could improve their choices. I can see the wheels turning in their minds: "I'll start that diet/online exercise class/go to the gym/lay off chips tomorrow."

The stumbling block is that all or nothing mentality. The "I'll gorge today and make up for it by starving tomorrow" kind of thinking, coupled with, "I blew it already, so what's the point?" They know they've done this to themselves. I did it as well.

What I tell them, around a mouthful of kale, is that I want to live to be 125, and they laugh. But based on all I've read and researched, I feel it's a realistic goal.

The secret to dieting is not to diet. What we all need to invest in is a lifestyle change. But it isn't all or nothing. A simple rule for living, and living well, is the 80/20 Rule.

The truth is, we're all on borrowed time. We only have one life to live. We all want to live longer—and live healthily—while maintaining a good quality of life. We want to be able to enjoy our lives and not burden others with avoidable illnesses or limitations. Life is challenging enough, and there is much we can't control: the weather, car accidents, others' mental states, the nasty waiter. But learning to be responsible and accountable for what you put in your body and how you prioritize your time is something you can control. In short, everything you do affects your health. Deciding to buy into your own health is one of the most important investments you'll ever make, and the currency is discipline.

"Okay," I can hear you say. "Stop right there. That's the problem. I don't have that. You know, the discipline."

Well, guess what? Discipline's really not the problem. The problem is the all or nothing mentality.

You need to live your life, not diet your way through life.

We are all a work in progress. We don't just arrive at health—we must always strive for it. I'm always trying out new strategies; moving to a plant-based diet and launching an intermittent fasting schedule are only two examples of how I switch it up. I make changes slowly but intentionally, aiming to land on the right decisions around eating and exercising most of the time and allowing myself to take a step back a minority of times. I follow a framework—the 80/20 Rule you'll hear more about in this book—to achieve my goals.

TAKE BABY STEPS

You're going to hear that a lot. Don't upend your life or your schedule to prove some point about being disciplined and able to get your life and health back on track in a month. If you've never been a runner, don't commit to five days at the gym and a circuit of 40 miles a week, or even five. That's setting yourself up for failure. Unless you're a professional athlete with a team of coaches, trainers, physiother-apists, and nutritionists, you won't have the kind of discipline to maintain a rigorous diet and exercise regime. Remember, we are all a work in progress. And taking baby steps makes sense. Success breeds success. If you take little steps and learn to recognize your victories, you're going to be more empowered to continue.

This brings me to two words: *can* and *should*. Too often, we tell ourselves we *should* choose to eat a bowl of braised greens, walnuts, and peppers, instead of fried steak and French fries. We say we *should* decide to get up at 5:30 in the morning and go to the gym be-fore that 8 o'clock power breakfast. But thinking in terms of *should* repeatedly backfires. *Should* sets you up to sabotage yourself. Who wants to be told what they *should* do? Even when it's you doing the telling, you kinda want to say no and rebel. Don't give yourself that opportunity. Instead, turn all that chatter about making choices into *can*. I *can* go to the gym. I *can* walk away from that second slice of cheesecake. Try it. It's amazing how much better you will get along with yourself!

FAILURE IS ALLOWED

This book gives you permission to fail. *I* give you permission. Better yet, I expect you to fail. You're going to mess up, and that's okay. Messing up means you tried. You can't mess up if you don't take some initiative and put yourself out there.

We all have the power to transform our health. But it is those of us who have already had their lives medicalized by heart disease, diabetes, cancer, or respiratory disease who are especially motivated to take on the challenge. We know what is at stake. But permission to fail is actually quite freeing. And if it makes you feel better, know that I mess up a lot. I just try not to mess up more than 20 percent of the time.

We all want to perform well and at our highest level, whether we are parents, or CEOs, or both. Our day-to-day lives matter. We can choose to make those days matter.

Unfortunately, so many don't make wise choices. According to the Centers for Disease Control (CDC), nearly 250,000 deaths from cardiovascular disease could be avoided every year if people made better decisions around diet and exercise. Overall, 20 to 40 percent of deaths from cardiovascular disease, chronic respiratory disease, and cancer could be prevented with better, more thoughtful diet and exercise.

The global cost of treating diabetes is expected to double to more than $2 trillion US by 2030. Yet 9 in 10 cases of Type 2 diabetes could be controlled by diet, exercise and other healthy lifestyle practices.

Much of the health crisis is preventable. I wrote this book so I could help you beat the ever-increasing odds of suffering a major illness or health event like a heart attack or stroke. It's hard to stay motivated when you *should* be sticking to a diet 100 percent of the time. Rather, you *can* eat well and exercise 80 percent of the time. You *can* learn to assess new information and add new activities or food choices, and try them out for a while—80 percent of the time.

My hope is that I can help you avoid health issues in the first place, and if you are already dealing with some, to learn how to effectively use diet and exercise to get on the path to improvement. I want you to invest in yourself now, so you can reap benefits for the rest of your life. I've transformed my health and my life, and this book will help you transform yours, too.

HOW TO USE THIS BOOK

This book is divided into four parts, with several sections in each. At the end of each part is a checklist that summarizes some of the key actions you can instantly apply to your routine and begin to take charge of your health.

You'll also find a simple framework—The Wheels of Health—that I use to get better control of my eating, exercise, sleep and mindful practices (see page 37).

To track your progress every day and every week, The Wheels of Health Daily Log is also included—you'll want to use it as a record of improvement, adding goals for the next day to help you reach your end goal. Sitting at lunch, or walking 30 minutes, for example. In the goals section, you might also add actions you'll be removing from your routine, such as scroll through my cell phone for one hour less than usual; invest in new running shoes; no sugar this week, or sleep eight hours. You decide. Make your own *can* statements. (See "The Wheels of Health Daily Log," page 172 for more.)

In addition, the book includes a recipe section with 30+ of my favorite plant-based recipes for inspiration and motivation to cook with less stress and enjoy healthy eating.

If you're looking for more inspiration, you can go to the website advicahealth.com/nevertoolatetobehealthy/ where I've added additional charts, and you can customize, print (if you like) and stuff them into the back of the book, or upload it to your electronic device.

The idea is to relax into the work ahead of you, because it's your life, and it will be good. Diet and exercise should not be this extra thing you do in your day. Gradually, over time, both will become integral parts of who you are. Food and exercise are just other parts of the day—fully integrated into your routine.

The book is designed for ease of use. You can dive in and out of the book and refresh your memory, or skip a section. I want this to be entertaining, informative, and approachable. If I achieve this, your life will be transformed. In transforming yourself, you will be leading by example and transforming those around you.

But remember, you don't have to do it all right now, and you don't even have to do it all. You can do it when you feel you're ready. And then, do it 80 percent of the time. Take those baby steps, chalk up a few successes, and look forward to more, not forgetting that there will be some setbacks. This is your life now. Not a diet.

Even if we say we don't like it, we live in a Type-A-gotta-be-perfect-100-percent-of-the-time world, and the stress is killing us. Seventy-five percent of people roll over and check their phones in the morning before looking out the window or greeting the person they're in bed with. Another 10 percent will have checked their phones in the middle of the night. (Hint: Write down "Don't look at the phone in the morning" in the goals section of your daily log!) This kind of stress is not something our bodies were designed to handle.

I used to be one of the 75 percent of people who check their cell phones before fully awake. I was one of those people who thought I was in shape. I thought I had the work-life balance sheet figured out, until I nearly ran out of time.

If you are reading this book, I figure you're efficient. Think of this as my way of saving you time. You don't need to figure all this out on your own. In terms of a learning curve, you can ride the steep line up. This book represents the 20 years of how I learned to live a better life. Think of the book you're reading as the condensed version. And I am glad to pass it on to you.

Life is only as rich and full as we perceive it to be. Your reality is shaped by you, your actions, and what you project to others. I've transformed my health completely. Today, not only am I the director of corporate health for a major insurance company while building a successful health business, but I've also qualified for the World Triathlon Championships for the last five years. I am stronger, fitter, and healthier now than I was when in college. The real gift is that today I am in a position to help others achieve their health and fitness goals, one baby step at a time.

There is no reason why we can't all lead healthy and active lives to 125.

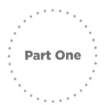
The
Early Years

Don't Drink and Die

"I think I'm gonna die," I said to the doctor in the med tent. There was no other way to describe what I was feeling. I stood shaking in a Mylar blanket, both cold and hot, feeling so incredibly weak. I felt beyond awful. Something was wrong.

The doctor glanced over. "You just ran 26.2 miles, man. You need to stretch out and rest. Here." He handed me a second blanket with the emblem for the Burlington Millennium Marathon on its tinseled front. I knew he was a marathoner himself. He passed me some Gatorade.

I took the drink, not sure I could get the cap off, but I was thirsty. Terribly thirsty. I had never been so thirsty. That day, May 31, 1999, was hot. Record-breaking hot at 30.3°C (nearly 87°F). Training all winter for this charity race meant I was prepared for the race but not prepared for the heat. I could take cold weather—rain, sleet, and fog—but a bright, clear, beautiful day with tons of sunlight was apparently about to do me in.

To make certain I didn't suffer heatstroke, I had made a heroic effort to stop at every water station along the way. I divvied up my fluids intake to water half the time and Gatorade the other half. The course was fairly flat. Burlington, Ontario, is not known for many heartbreak hills, and I had run other marathons. Considering the heat, my time was decent, finishing in just under four hours, perhaps a little slower than usual, but I kept pushing myself. Along the route, I chatted with other runners—young men and women, older men and women, a handful of real old-timers, and guys like me, thirtysomethings with jobs and kids and spouses. It felt like a good race, a good pace, and I made sure I kept hydrated. I chatted with the support people handing out orange wedges and drinks. I wasn't incoherent, and no red flags went up.

Now, though, with the race over and bundled in mylar, my entire body was cramping, and I felt weak and sick. Not really nauseated, but dizzy and somehow outside of myself, a horribly surreal sensation. All I knew was that I was dying.

I returned to the tent.

The doctor sent me away a second time, dismissing my condition as just the worry of another athlete needing to recuperate after a heavy run. After outlining again that I had just run a marathon, he took my blood pressure and heart rate and, although it was a bit elevated, he told me to go home. What was wrong with me was not on most medical professionals' radar at the time, and that included this doctor's.

But I knew I was in a grave situation. After the race, when people asked me how I felt, I said, "I feel like I'm dying," and they'd nod in sympathy. They had no idea I was serious.

Just the same, I didn't want people looking at me.

The course ended at a large indoor-outdoor pavilion, a beautiful spot on the shore of Lake Ontario. I laid down in the grass on the other side of all the activity, where no one could see me, and tried to get my bearings, tried to will myself to feel better. My seven-year-old son, Tim, was playing beside me and at one point asked, "Dad, are you okay?"

Of course, I told him I was fine. I was in shape, fit. I just needed to slug down another drink, and I certainly didn't want him worrying about me.

Maybe the doctor was right. As an athlete, I was used to blocking out pain or discomfort. If I felt something going wrong on the run, I couldn't remember. But I definitely did not feel like myself.

Then something went sideways. I heaved myself up and somehow made it into the medical tent a third time. This time I sat on one of the beds. Several marathoners were hooked to IVs to replenish fluids. Maybe that's what I needed. I was dehydrated. I was still so thirsty. My brain felt fuzzy. I remember the doctor took my pulse, checked my heart rate and temperature, and told me again, kindly, to just go home and rest.

But I knew something was really wrong. I told my wife, Barb, to go get the truck because I didn't think I'd make it to the parking lot. I couldn't think straight. I knew my four-year-old son, Matt, had a recital later that afternoon that I wanted to attend, yet I felt compelled to follow the doctor's instructions to rest.

The plan was to go to Matt's recital and then head home; we had enough time to do both. Instead, by the time Barb was back with the truck, I knew I wouldn't be able to make it to the recital. Instead, I asked her to drop Matt off and then come back to get me so I could have more time to recuperate. Tim stayed, sitting next to me while I lay in misery. I finally asked the doctor to call an ambulance. With some reluctance, he called, but I have no recollection of how long it took them to get to us. I just remember climbing into the ambulance with Tim at my side.

Later, I found out that Barb had driven Matt to meet his grandma at the recital and was on her way back to the race tent to check up on me. She passed an ambulance with its sirens on, speeding the other way. Little did she know that I was in it, heading to the hospital.

I can remember being in the back of the ambulance with Tim. Relieved I was under medical care, I allowed my mind to relax and drift. I don't remember anything else until I woke up from my coma one week later.

DR. 'KEEP 'EM ALIVE' CLIVE

By the time I arrived at the hospital in Burlington, it had taken 11 doctors and nurses to restrain me, holding me down because I was convulsing so badly. My wife, who had followed in our truck with our daughter (still young enough to be in a booster seat) and my brother, remembers a code blue call, which means an emergency like cardiac arrest or respiratory failure. An MRI of my brain showed swelling.

> I was dying. The emergency team sedated me until they could figure out what was going on with my body. I was 36 years old, in good shape, ate right. No history of heart trouble. And yet, my body was shutting down. Kidney failure came next.

I was transferred by ambulance from Burlington to a bigger hospital in nearby Hamilton, Ontario, and shifted to the care of Dr. 'Keep 'em Alive' Clive. A CAT scan was performed, and Dr. Clive arrived at a diagnosis. As my family watched over me during the week I was in a coma, he figured out what had nearly killed me: exercise-associated hyponatremia (EAH). Initially described in 1985 in endurance athletes, EAH used to be considered quite rare and something that only struck ultramarathoners running in extreme heat. (An ultramarathon is any distance longer than the traditional 26-mile marathon length, most often in the realm of 50 to 150 miles.)

Then two charity marathoners died in the summer of 2002. Both women passed away within two days of their races, their brains swollen and their organs failing. But I was sick in 1999, and the public and much of the medical community was not yet aware of the dire consequences of drinking too many fluids.

It turns out that drinking excessive amounts of water can lead to low sodium. My blood had literally become diluted, and all that extra water overwhelmed my kidneys' ability to excrete the liquid. Perspiration also reduces sodium. Because I lost sodium through sweating and then drank too much water during the marathon, the sodium content of my blood dropped dramatically. Then, because of this critical imbalance of sodium, my brain swelled with fluid.

Dr. Clive was able to get me stabilized and take me off the ventilator; I came out of the coma to see the faces of my worried family members. To this day, I still have very little memory of what happened in those minutes after the race. All I know for sure is that I am very lucky to be alive, and I have Dr. Clive to thank. I became part of a new, but sobering, statistic: 11 to 15 percent of endurance athletes suffer from hyponatremia, with 1 percent of cases proving fatal.

The doctors who initially saw me had told Barb I had a less than 10 percent chance of survival because, after a week on full life support,

I had not come out of my coma. The medical team was also very worried that if I did come out of my coma my brain would be damaged.

HEALING AND SELF-REFLECTION

I spent the whole summer recuperating. Recovering from hyponatremia is far different than recovering from dehydration. In severe heatstroke, with rest and fluids, most patients can be back on their feet in a week. Even with milder cases of hyponatremia, recovery is much slower. In my case, I was weak, disoriented. I ended up gaining my strength back at our summer cottage, and starting the process of self-reflection: What should I be doing differently? What should I change in my life? How should I change? I didn't know what to do. And back then, I had no idea there would be other health issues I would be facing even after recovery.

Plus, I was stressed. I had just started a business that May and now had to take three months off to recover. It doesn't take an expert to know this was no way to get a business off the ground. The entrepreneur in me bit my nails and pushed forward. I had no choice. But walking from our home's front door to the kids' bus stop was exhausting. I had to improve my stamina, my mental state, my life. This wasn't optional.

That summer I faced some hard truths. I was 36—True. I was in peak condition—False. I cared about my health—True. I knew how to get better—False. I loved my family—True. I knew how to live as long as possible—False. My systems weren't as sharp as they could have been. Even going into the race, I knew I hadn't eaten properly, that something wasn't quite right with my body. In short, I knew I could do better to reach my health goals, or at least achieve the vision I saw of myself: fit, healthy, and living a long and productive life. Something, clearly, was off.

What I realized then was that something had been off my whole life. Yes, I was busy raising kids, helping run a house, being an involved dad. But I was also running a business, sometimes multiple businesses, training, drinking, and eating not-so-healthy food at not-so-healthy times. I wasn't getting enough sleep, and I certainly wasn't investing in giving myself a shot at a long and healthy life. Nearly dying showed me, up close, how fleeting and fragile life is. Before my race, I felt I could continue on the path that had worked for years and 'exercise' myself to good health. But that wasn't the case—I was ignoring the other critical parts of health, including stress management, nutrition, and rest.

This was merely the *start* of my health journey. Several years later, I would visit a doctor who would perform a multitude of tests, the results of which pointed to dire conclusions. It was only then that I truly began the shift in my approach to leading a lifestyle, a lifestyle that embraced and practiced all the tenets of healthy living daily. I was fit, but I needed to make changes to get healthy.

THE ALARM WENT OFF TWICE

It wasn't until I was nearly 50 years old that I had my true wake-up call and had to permanently change my ways. After my collapse at the marathon and my coma, followed by months of rehab and relearning—how to walk to the post office box without becoming totally fatigued, for instance—I thought I was making the required effort to achieve good health. I continued to exercise and work out, but I would be lying if I said I was doing everything right, and that included instituting a change in my eating habits. It was easy to compartmentalize the hyponatremia as a freak occurrence due to the oversaturation of fluids and the lack of sodium in my body. I never fully connected the dots that my general health and lifestyle might have set the stage to literally drown myself.

Fast forward a decade and I'm in my doctor's office for my annual executive medical, expecting good results, when he sits me down for a serious talk. Dr. Randy is a tall, fit guy in his 50s and the medical director of a successful executive medical practice in Ontario. I heard the faint ring of alarm bells going off again.

"Kevin, I have to be honest with you. You're prediabetic. You have high blood pressure and high cholesterol," Dr. Randy said.

"But don't worry," he continued. "That's normal for people your age." He then drew a graph on his clipboard, indicating how the conditions would get worse every year based on how people age. In fact, he assured me that it was normal for a person at my stage of life to start going on meds. It was to be expected. In this context, 'normal' wasn't making me feel particularly at ease.

"We need to put you on meds," he reiterated, leveling his gaze at me. He wanted to start me on prescriptions right away to reduce my cholesterol, high blood pressure and high sugar levels. I was also still overweight, despite being a regular runner. I knew that delivering this kind of news was all in a day's work for him, but I pushed back.

"Give me three months," I said. "You're going to see a dramatic difference."

He looked skeptical, and I couldn't blame him. "You've basically been abusing your body all these years," he said. "It's not like it's just going to turn around in three months." But he agreed to do another blood panel in 90 days.

I was determined. It was as if a lightbulb had just gone on in my head. It wasn't that I didn't trust my doctor—I did. I'd been going to him for several years and had every reason to believe he was right.

PERMISSION TO CHANGE

Today, 22 years later, I am in a continuous process of staying healthy—and loving it. Taking care of my health and helping others manage theirs is a passion of mine that I could not have predicted back then.

I changed from *thinking* I was healthy to *being* healthy. There are a lot of people out there who don't eat right or exercise, but there are many others who do or think they do. I was one of those people. People with the right mental attitude, who schedule time for exercise and attend to family life and friends, in an attempt to achieve that sweet spot on the teeter-totter of work-life balance.

What I want to hand off to you are the big take-aways from my life of living well.

If you follow the basic tenets of this book, you will wake up one day and realize that living a life mindful of health is just an integral part of each day. That paying attention to diet, exercise, sleep, and mental agility are so woven into the fabric of your day, so much a part of the enjoyment of your waking hours, that your healthy lifestyle is at once transparently routine and yet offers true joy and self-confidence.

None of this will happen overnight. It certainly didn't happen overnight for me. You are getting the benefit of this book, the Kevin Brady condensed version, and will reap the benefits without the tedium of trial and error. I want to give you permission to make a healthy change, and that's a small step right there. You don't have to do it all at once.

Having the proper mindset is the key to any process, and this *is* a process. You must decide you want this, that you want to wake up one day and *not* notice that nearly everything you do, from what you put in your mouth to how you move your body to decisions about when to go to bed to practicing some kind of mental exercise, is all driven by a fundamental commitment to health. Rather, this will just be your life. I know it sounds like a lot. A lot of change. And many people are resistant to that.

> **Here's what I learned, and you will read this again and again: You don't have to do it all at once. That kind of change is not sustainable.**

Some changes we can't control, like a debilitating accident or a job dependent on a relocation. Having a baby instantly changes you into a parent. But the choices that will help us live better, more productive, healthy lives are ones we can control. We can get into a rhythm of self-sabotage or forming bad habits. Take, for example, using food as emotional comfort—like grabbing a bag of chips or a big bowl of ice cream to fill a void or soothe a stressful time. Recognizing the behavior or pattern in itself can help drive things around on a road to better health.

This is your chance to truly make a difference in your own life and life expectancy and spend a little more time on this planet with those you love.

SHIFTING EXPECTATIONS

In order to be successful and keep making progress, we need to agree to shift expectations. All these diets that promise five pounds off in a week, protein shakes promising pounds of muscle, or a new exercise routine that seems tantalizingly easy and short—they all raise expectations about what we can accomplish in a (usually) short amount of time.

The truth is you can't fast track your health. However, you *can* see improvement in a couple of months. You might feel better by going to the gym almost immediately. I'm not saying the body does not immediately respond to good care, because it does. What I'm saying is that the expectation of 'this X plan works now, and then I'll drop it when results are achieved' never, ever works. Let's say you want to lose 15 pounds, so you go on some diet of the moment. One of two internal scenarios can play out as 12 lbs come off: 1) I'll just stop now and hope I can maintain it; 2) I will try to maintain the regime even though I hate it/it's boring/the food is gross/I have no energy, time, commitment.

Twelve-step programs offer us this adage: Expectations are premeditated resentments. Think of the last person you resented because they didn't live up to some expectation you had of them, or from them. So, if you set up unreasonably high expectations for yourself that can only be met for a short time under pristine conditions, guess whom you're going to resent?

You.

Diets and wellness programs often use magical thinking as leverage in a world where it seems that expecting something to happen might make it happen.

It doesn't. Expecting something to happen won't make it happen.

We also have an unrealistic tendency to assume that fulfilled expectations translate to happiness. If I reach this goal, meet this expectation, I will be happy, so goes the equation. Not true. You may fulfill an expectation, such as starting a company, and end up being very unhappy. Smaller expectations tend to lead to great happiness. I expect to share information about health and exercise with my grown children, for example, and so a recipe swap brings a lot of joy. Those kinds of expectations are achievable because we have already experienced the results, or at least can anticipate them.

Expectations set too high, without good reasons for those expectations, result in disappointment. An executive might say to herself in the exhilaration of just joining a gym: "I will get to the gym five days this week," even though she knows she has seven meetings set up and will be out of town for three days of that first week. She's already defeated. The chances she'll even go the second week are pretty slim.

USE THE 80/20 RULE

The 80/20 Rule provides a framework for setting up nutrition and exercise goals. It reflects the idea that we are all a work in progress and that we are all continually working to improve our health, slowly, one goal at a time, with clear intentions. So I strive to make the right decisions around eating and exercising 80 percent of the time and allow myself to take a step back, have pizza at a party, skip a workout, 20 percent of the time. If I eat 10 portions of food in one day, two are allowed to be 'off-limits' if the other eight are balanced and nutritionally sound. Here's my big secret: I still eat Doritos once in a while. Love 'em.

What you can do is set parameters for yourself: the 80/20 Rule. This allows you to carry some expectations and therefore set goals, but gives you a reprieve from self-flagellation. If you are moving down that path of healthy living 80 percent of the time you will, by definition, be successful 100 percent of the time. Even when you screw up. Because you will. We all do. I certainly did and continue to do so.

Knowing you can step off the path 20 percent of the time, regroup, have that bowl of chips, or take a walk and not a run, helps you keep expectations low and successes high. Success really does breed success. Nothing will keep you motivated and focused like success. So, if failure is built into the formula for success, you are already ahead. Failure is a part of any worthwhile endeavor. Adhering to the 80/20 Rule is like incorporating planned obsolescence—in this case, it's planned failure. Another healthy way to frame this mindset is to realize you are already planning to deviate from the ideal.

A DIFFERENT WAY TO THINK ABOUT GOALS

When people talk about goals and goal setting, they are usually describing three basic types of objectives, where time, focus, or topic represent the endgame. The problem with most diets and healthy living regimens is that setting goals nearly always revolves around the first two targets: time and focus. The time frame is short, 'Get into shape fast!' and the focus is on one giant change like NEVER EAT SUGAR AGAIN, or RUN EVERY DAY, or, as you scrape your plate of leftover prime rib, I WILL GO VEGAN TOMORROW.

However, the third aim—topic—is more indicative of personal goals, such as eating healthier or exercising better. If your overarching goal is to live to 125 and live well, then the objectives to meet that goal are the baby steps.

Athletes and sports enthusiasts like me tend to look at setting goals with three different objectives: performance, processs, and outcome. Though both performance and outcome are important—we certainly want to lift more weight, run farther, sleep well, and then be able to measure those outcomes—it is process that's the focus of this book.

The 80/20 Rule has many constructive and powerful applications. It wouldn't work in brain surgery or space flight, but you're not operating on anyone while you eat, and with rare exceptions, I don't see many of you commanding a rocket ship. So the stakes are already lower, as are the expectations. Over time, however, as you, your family, friends, doctors, and colleagues see the changes in your body and mind, those expectations will actually evaporate. In their place will come a far more powerful realization: You are now living a healthy life.

And then all sorts of changes emerge. You start to see your friends taking an interest in how you transformed yourself. Your family members may begin to follow your lead. Colleagues at work will find your stories of new recipes fascinating or a new mindfulness technique you discovered absolutely riveting. There will be, of course, a lot of teasing you may have to endure, but in the long run, you will be leading by example. You will be the living, breathing proof that a healthy life is a process of discovery, and that process is worthwhile, with benefits both personal and profound.

This book will help you get there. All you need to do is shift your mindset to the following: My health is important, and I need to take care of the one body I have. Then ratchet those expectations down a notch or two. Instead of throwing yourself into some routine you can never sustain, take baby steps. Give yourself permission to fail. Get back on track when you 'screw up,' and most importantly, enjoy the ride.

The wheels are turning. We're getting ready to start down a new road to health.

Getting In Tune with Wellness

I was not always on this road myself. I didn't grow up in some super-fit, granola-crunching, stop-watch record-holding family that took health to the next level. Looking back, I had a fairly typical upbringing—raised in a pretty middle class home—and my family's attitude to health was educated, but not focused. Like a lot of mothers in the '60s and '70s, mine paid special attention to diet and nutrition. I remember her always reading articles about food and vitamins in magazines like *Good Housekeeping* and *Chatelaine*. From the time I was very young, my mom suffered from chronic pneumonia and searched for possible preemptive solutions—she tried massive doses of vitamin C, ginger tea, heating pads, and vitamin E supplements.

Even though she was hospitalized a number of times, I didn't know how serious it was until I grew older. I can remember being just seven years old and having to go stay with family friends since I was the youngest of the four kids in our family. One of the reasons it took years for me to realize the seriousness of my mom's condition was because my parents never brought any drama to the table. Her illness remained a difficult topic we didn't discuss very often.

There was a pattern that developed around her illness. She'd be gone for several weeks. Then one day, I'd return home from school and my mother would be in the kitchen, resuming her routines around the house and, in the weeks that followed, spending time researching the newest health craze. Back then, it was eating saccharin instead of sugar and drinking skim or powdered milk instead of whole milk (for the record, I hated skim milk powder!). Spreading margarine instead of butter on pancakes. I am not sure we ever drank Tang, but if it promised to deliver more vitamin C, we could have it.

MY HEALTH GROWING UP

As a kid, I rebelled against jumping on the nutrition bandwagon. I did not want to swallow a giant vitamin C tablet every morning while my mom looked on. The focus on eating well, however, was little more than taking a vitamin pill. In terms of food, our meals were quite simple. I wasn't eating salads every night and having health shakes for breakfast, but I grew up in a house that made nutrition a priority. It wasn't at the top of the list, but a balanced diet was at least *on* the list, maybe somewhere in the middle. Both my parents are English-Irish, so our meals and food choices were typical and traditional, with meat and two or three small servings of vegetables coupled with a starch like rice or potatoes or turnips.

We were served dessert every night: kid heaven.

If you were to question my mom on serving healthy meals to her family, she would have said she was doing her best with the information she had. But people didn't know then what they know now.

We ate according to guidelines from a food pyramid that hadn't changed in decades, eating food processed with salt and increasing amounts of sugar. We consumed fillers, dyes, pesticides—in short, a diet that led much of the general public to insulin resistance, diabetes, coronary heart disease, and obesity. So, though our diet wasn't *bad*, it was typical. If my mom had access to the information we have now, with the wisdom of hindsight, she would have made all of us eat organic salads and more plant-based meals, and trotted us off to school after forcing us to drink vegetable and fruit morning shakes.

In terms of exercise, we were a physically active family. We participated in many different sports, and we grew up swimming, playing hockey, baseball, football. I was a lifeguard in high school and college and participated in all the sports at school: football, hockey, basketball; plus, I swam competitively in both high school and college. No matter what the season, I was moving. From football season, I'd go into hockey and from hockey to swimming. In high school, I also rowed competitively. One year, a bunch of us traveled to the Canadian championships, and a few went on to the Olympics. Though I was never at that level of elite athleticism, that ethos appealed to me and I could appreciate the hard work, the discipline, and the payoff of being in shape.

Though I played sports and appreciated exercising, I wasn't up at 4 a.m. obsessing over my time or gnawing on boiled chicken breasts. I would run because I had to in order to be in shape for rowing, but I didn't really enjoy it. And, of course, I partied like most college students, rationalizing my misadventures as many do as part of the 'work hard, play hard' mentality.

In college, watching the Grey Cup, the Canadian equivalent to the Super Bowl, was basically a license to get up at 9 in the morning and start drinking, and the residents would be in full party mode. Pregame festivities, a halftime show and another excuse to hang out with friends all whetted an appetite for a lot of alcohol, bad food, and sometimes bad behavior.

I was a normal Canadian kid with no superhuman desire to be a health guru. I carried typical family attitudes toward nutrition and exercise right into college, where they then deteriorated somewhat. Let's just say there were a lot of burgers and pizzas.

THANK GOD I MET BARB

When Barb and I married, I cleaned up my partying ways, and when we started having children, we ate what we thought was a healthy diet. Meat, starch, vegetables, closing with a flourish of dessert. We used food to celebrate the small moments, like when our kids started playing sports. We'd celebrate every game with a Peanut Buster

Parfait. Every week. Every. Single. Week. Dairy Queen became just a part of the weekly game routine.

When Tim, our youngest child, was a baby and we lived in Calgary, I would go biking and put his baby seat on the back of my bike. We had just moved to Calgary so I could assume my position as a senior manager of a major insurance company. I began going to the YMCA and met people who seemed to be pretty hard-core fitness advocates in a variety of disciplines. One guy was on the national ski team and asked if I was a mountain biker.

My "Sure" may have come out a little too fast.

The next thing I knew I was invited—and feeling under some pressure—to an all-day event where cyclists performed laps on the mountain in relays. Picture this: Ten people on a team each take a leg of the route. Now, I was from Ontario, with fairly flat roadways when you consider other places in Canada. It's like a giant plate and nothing like the mountainous terrain of Calgary. The truth was, I didn't even have a real mountain bike.

I showed up to the race with my hybrid, a cross between a road bike and a mountain bike, and my stretchy pants. Everyone else was in dense, padded spandex gear and clippings. They were all die-hard mountain bikers, and none of them were hiding their alarm when they saw my running shoes. Worse? There was a baby seat on the back of my bike. I had 'novice' stamped all over me.

I scaled up the mountain, pedaling on my substandard, domesticated bike in my inappropriate shoes, and every time I rocketed down the mountain I'd wipe out.

But these guys were great. I became an instant celebrity, and they all gave me credit for the attempt. I was so touched. I ended up skiing with this group over the next few winters as well. I realized I had to start doing more exercise on a regular basis if I wanted to keep up with them.

Even though I hated running in college, it was fast, easy, cheap, and required no special gear, so I kept at it. I ran long and hard, and was eating 'well,' but I wasn't focused on eating better as a lifestyle choice, a means to a better, stronger, healthier me.

Looking back on that period in my 30s, I weighed 240 pounds and was just thinking I needed to take my running to the next level. One of my friends in Calgary was turning 40, and he wanted to run a marathon. Would I run it with him? Sounded good. I'd been keeping up with shorter runs and thought I was in pretty good shape. We trained, and I joined a group called the Running Room, which basically helps you progress, teaching you how to run a marathon in 20 weeks. Although I was running long distances and getting the mental and physical discipline down, I was still not focused on food and nutrition and the fuel I was putting in my body.

"I CAN TRAIN MYSELF OUT OF ANYTHING"

Though I worked hard to get my body in pretty decent shape, I was under the false impression that I could, if I worked hard enough, train myself out of any health issue. In other words, I would always have good health as long as I pushed hard to exercise. When I was first married, and my kids were young, I really thought I had it all figured out. (Like I did about everything else, too!) Though I was training for a marathon, I wasn't exercising at the level I am now. That said, exercise was my focus, and food was not even a blip on my radar. I ate what I wanted, partied some (which I still do), but never made the basic and very real link between performance and nutrition. I didn't realize then that good diet, good sleep and low stress were equally as important.

That first marathon was in Kelowna, British Columbia, in 1996. I ran two more in London, Ontario, before my collapse in 1999 in Burlington. That first one in Kelowna had me hooked. I loved the mental state it put me into, and I loved the feeling of completion. But most of all, it turned out I loved to run. I made it work, with some help from my son. When Tim was young and I was training, he would climb onto his little bike with training wheels and pedal along with me as I ran. This turned an activity I was ambivalent about into something I looked forward to, and I slowly began to realize the power of success. The more I ran, the more I liked to run.

We moved back to Ontario, and by that time I was training regularly for marathons. Tim would be out on his little bike pedaling fast, and I'd be jogging along at a good pace. We had a lot of fun. I'd run for three hours with him pedaling along beside me, and I'd stop at a Tim Hortons and get a coffee or water and keep running.

Though I was modeling an active lifestyle, I was not modeling good eating habits.

We'd have junk food in the house within easy reach. The kids even remember traveling down to the U.S. to ski and race, and on the way home we'd stop at a gas station and we'd all go in and order pizza, hot dogs, and subs. They still laugh because I would buy a 12-pack of Krispy Kreme doughnuts or Twinkies for the car ride home. That's more than two pastries apiece, and now it makes me positively shudder to think about it. Often in processed foods like that, there are so many chemical additives and preservatives that the food lasts for 10 years. Okay, I might be exaggerating, but not by much. That test where they put a fast-food hamburger in a glass jar and a homemade hamburger made with healthy ingredients in another jar reinforces my point. The fast-food hamburger looks tasty weeks later, and the homemade one starts looking wonky after just 24 hours. In this case, trust me when I say we should be going for wonky.

To be fair, we were young, with young kids, and often on a tight budget. We bought food we thought was healthy enough and affordable. We became really good at finding ways to cook and eat tomatoes, beans, pasta, and rice. We did what we believed to be the best with what we had.

In all probability, I was just like many of you. I was health informed but not health conscious. I was exercising, but not at peak performance. I was focused on work, not connections. And my mind was filled with future to-dos, not with the present.

The moral of the story is this: If I can clean up my act, you can do it, too. You've already taken steps to do so. You picked up this book, right? You're ready for change.

CHECKLIST: STRATEGIES FOR CHANGE

Here's the first of several checklists throughout the book, intended to highlight key points from every preceding section. All these checklists act as living, breathing documents, meant to offer a means to help make small adjustments and keep you moving forward. Feel free to add your own strategies, too.

- Schedule an annual health assessment.
- Get your full blood and urine panel done annually.
- Live by the 80/20 Rule.
- Take baby steps.
- Practice a daily exercise routine.

Part Two

The
Wheels
of Health

The Keys to Your Health Transformation

In this section of the book, we're going to cover basic components of the Wheels of Health, as you progress toward a healthier, more vibrant you. Consider *eating right, exercising regularly, sleeping well, and learning to be more mindful* as the spokes of your wheel. When these are all aligned properly, they will keep the wheel turning and moving forward toward building better health and a better life, community, and sense of well-being. The goal is to keep all four wheels in balance. If one wheel is out of balance, it affects all the other wheels.

When one wheel gets out of whack, it affects everything else. Keeping the four wheels, at least roughly aligned, is your roadmap to peak performance or, more simply, better health. As you balance these components, you'll want to keep the 80/20 Rule I outlined earlier in mind.

To fully appreciate how all these areas overlap, think for a moment about the choices you make when you're feeling exhausted and sleep deprived. Are you more likely to reach for the sugar-coated doughnut, a bag of deliciously salty chips, or take the time to make a healthy salad or shake? Chances are, like most people, when tired or pressed for time you'll opt for the quick sugar high or sodium boost. It's okay—you're human. You're tired, so you reach for the I-don't-have-to-think-about-it snack. It's just one example of how something we don't pay attention to can affect us; more specifically, how sleep winds up being critical to making good eating choices. But how do we know what to eat? How do we decide which diet to start? No carbs? Some carbs? No gluten? No sugar?

It's no wonder we're confused. In the last decade alone, there have been an endless number of studies on nutrition and even more books on diet, each espousing some new 'secret' to weight loss and better health.

How do you wade through all this information? How do you decide what and when and *how* to eat?

Think of the wheels of a car. You need to keep them balanced, or the car doesn't run well. You might even lose control! The wheels are dependent on one another, so if one is out of balance it affects the others. For example, if you're stressed, you'll likely not sleep well. If you don't sleep well, then you won't have the energy to exercise or exercise at peak performance. In addition, if you're tired, you'll be looking for quick energy, likely opting for the unhealthy sweet snack and a sugar rush. After 15 minutes, you'll crash, and the cycle will begin again.

Bottom line? Keep those wheels aligned!

THE WHEEL OF HEALTH ASSESSMENT

The Wheel of Health is an assessment tool you can use to determine the areas of your life that are in or out of balance. It helps you better understand which part of your life might need more attention. For simplicity, we use 1 wheel instead of 4 wheels to mark our progress. The Wheel, shown here, has 5 levels (with level 1 indicating dissatisfaction/needs improvement in that area and level 5 indicating satisfaction with your health in that area). In each quadrant, draw an "X" or a star where you score yourself on a level of 1 to 5.

I recommend setting goals for yourself on how to improve and maintain each quadrant of your health. Use an "O" to mark where you want to be on the Wheel. Ask yourself what small habits you can change along the way, or what type of support you may need to achieve your goal. You can repeat this exercise in a few months time and see if you have improved upon your initial rank. Initially, the exercise might show that you require big improvements, for example, in the areas of Exercise and Mindfulness. Ultimately, you want to have the 4 parts of the Wheel all balanced in the upper 5th level.

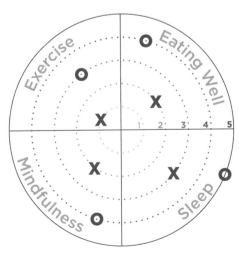

Rank Your Wheel of Health

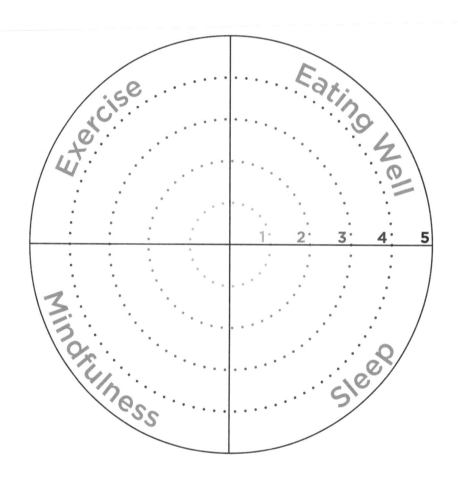

Eating Well

Despite my very real brush with death in my late 30s, it wasn't until that routine annual checkup with Dr. Randy nearly 20 years later that I began to change my eating habits.

The realization that I wasn't as healthy as I could be, that I was, in fact, prediabetic with high blood pressue and high cholesterol, finally flipped the switch. I was not okay with taking meds. I could not accept that this was normal for someone my age. I would not adopt the protocol my doctor was advising, even if he had every reason to believe I could not 'fix' my health with a significant change in my diet.

Maybe it was because of my work in the health and wellness field, or just my general bullheadedness or, more likely, a combination of both, but I spent the next month completely changing my typical North American diet. Dr. Randy was surprised to see me only a month later when I turned up 60 days early, eager to have my blood panels done again. He told me not to expect to see a big difference in such a short time.

A few days later, I got a call: "You're my star patient! All your levels have dropped significantly and, in fact, you are in the low range on all readings now. What have you been doing?"

Now, I don't want you to think that overnight I developed some kind of superhuman ability to suddenly change all my eating habits. But I was definitely focused and determined to make a difference, and began to turn my health around. And I did, with shakes, supplements, and a different attitude toward food. I also didn't do just one thing. I switched it up. Here's a secret: I still switch it up all the time.

Remember, I grew up eating the most basic North American diet imaginable. Every meal was just a slightly different mix of meat, a small helping of vegetables, and a sizeable portion of some form of white starch. I never thought twice about eating any other way for most of my life. But when I was handed this challenge from my doctor—though I don't think he viewed it in those terms—I developed a morning routine I stick with to this day, devised a supplement plan based on my medical tests, and began substituting better foods for those I knew were going to kill me.

SHAKE IT OFF

I started by simply doing away with my usual breakfast of yogurt, fruit, granola, and sometimes toast and peanut butter. On weekends I would splurge and have eggs and bacon. Now, with the threat of pills being added to my daily regime, I downed a healthy shake I would make in my blender. Throwing in whatever I could find—usually an abundance of fruits and veggies, seeds like chia or flax, some protein powder, and other nutrients—I learned to look forward to my thick, greenish shake, and it has become part of the routine I use to this day. I have been doing my signature shake as part of my morning routine for several years now and I believe it is the very best way to start the day. Even though I typically have other servings of fruit and vegetables during the day, when it isn't possible I feel good about the fact that I consumed my full requirement that morning.

But don't just take my word for it. Try it! (See recipe for The Wilson Shake, on page 126.) Giving the body something good to work with can kick-start healing. According to The Center for Nutrition Studies, "When the requirements of health are appropriately provided, the self-healing mechanisms of the body attempt to restore and/or optimize health. Your body's ability to do this is only limited by your inherent constitution (genetics) and the amount of use and abuse that has taken place." Once I started consistently putting good food into my body, it responded and triggered its own natural healing mechanisms, which resulted in the improved levels my doctor reported only a month later.

The shake first involved frozen fruit and whey protein, but it has evolved significantly over the last few years. I now use frozen organic fresh fruits and vegetables, plant-based protein powder, chia or flax seed, and alternating different powders, such as spirulina, maca, or other proteins, combined with two liters of water. You can use the recipe on page 126, but I encourage you to do your own experiments because there is no one-size-fits-all shake. Tweak it to fit your taste buds. But a good blender, blending wand, or Vitamix is essential.

I am not the only one who has enjoyed my shakes. My dog, Wilson, a white Westiepoo who was about 11 years old at the time, would watch me curiously, waiting for me to share the dregs of the shake with him. Wilson died at the ripe old age of 18, and my family has a theory that the shake helped him live such a long life. Every morning, Wilson would beg and whine for his daily share of my plant-based morning shake! He loved it so much, we've dubbed the drink The Wilson Shake. But seriously, the takeaway here is how quickly the body responds to good input and good nutrition.

How quickly? Thirty days.

WHAT IF THERE WAS A PILL FOR THAT?

I am not a saint. I did not give up sugar or chips entirely. Remember my ongoing love for Doritos? I just added more good ingredients than bad and made a consistent habit out of making sure I consumed my daily servings of fruits and vegetables every morning in the form of my shake.

Starting your day this way is akin to the idea of paying yourself first when it comes to saving money. You're doing something positive and healthy for yourself first thing in the morning. This is a great, regular habit to get into. So, if you find yourself later in the day at an office birthday party gathering and someone passes you a paper plate with a slice of devil's food cake on it—you may decide to pass on it, or you may choose to enjoy it without guilt because you know you've already fed your body a huge serving of nutrients just hours before. This is the 80/20 Rule in action.

People are always looking for a magic pill. What if I could develop a pill that would significantly reduce the sickness, disease, and illness in the world? If I could do that, I'd be a billionaire many times over. But it is worth thinking about.

What if I could develop a pill that would:

- reduce obesity
- eliminate Type 2 diabetes
- lower blood pressure
- eliminate cardiovascular disease
- reduce heart attacks
- reduce dementia
- reduce the effects of, and slow the progression of, Alzheimer's disease
- reduce inflammatory diseases
- reduce arthritis
- reduce body fat

In addition, what if the pill also left you feeling amazing and with the vigor to tackle every day with the energy of a 25 year old? And your friends and family were desperate to find the bottle?

Well, I have the 'pill' that does all of that— only, of course, it's not a pill.

EATING BY THE 80/20 RULE

This is another strategy I use to commit to eating well, as it allows me to enjoy life while still improving and paying attention to my health. Obviously, the ideal from a health standpoint would be to watch every single thing I eat 24/7. Living by the 80/20 Rule means that I try to eat and be healthy 80 percent of the time. It also allows me to enjoy life, enjoy good food, drink, *and* plunge my hand into a bag of chips once in a while. For me, this typically happens on weekends.

I know this is different from what you've read before. My health advice is not what you'd come across in most popular health or diet blogs. Everyone is busy espousing one way or type of eating.

Social media may insist that you maintain a cult-like devotion to whatever brand of health, eating, or fitness regime is the current flavor of the month. I say, toss that idea out the window along with the package of Twinkies you no longer need.

Just be certain you know what healthy eating is so that 80 percent counts! I realized that a few years ago when I thought I was eating healthily 80 percent of the time. However, since I've embarked on this path, I've learned that what I thought was good food for my body was, in fact, not that good at all. What I try to focus on now are minor improvements that add up over time. For example, a couple of years ago, I gave up dairy. The year before that, I started going to bed earlier so I could have a longer night's sleep. I didn't do both in the same week. Or in the same month. Over the years, I've made many small changes that now add up to a much healthier lifestyle.

Over time, I've modified my diet and moved the needle in a better direction, so now I'm consuming healthy food 80 percent of the time rather than 50 percent of the time. So yes, the 80/20 Rule allows for flexibility, but you have to be loyal and committed to that 80 percent.

Studies have shown that the standard North American diet is comprised of 60 percent ultra-processed foods and only 5 to 10 percent plants, fruits and vegetables. In fact, flipping the statistics so that the large majority of what we eat are plants, vegetables and whole foods should be the norm, and would positively impact common health conditions like diabetes, high blood pressure, heart disease, and cancers. The only person keeping you from changing that typical diet is you. But you shouldn't just suddenly go to a plant-based diet or even a primarily plant-based diet in a week. Do it in stages. Over time, you'll come to think that highly processed food tastes like cardboard.

I think a reason people fail to reach their health goals is that if they get off track, they figure they've blown it, so they revert to old habits. It really is okay to 'cheat' once in a while if you make a healthy change for the majority of the time. After all, you're doing 80 percent better than you were before. Trust me. I'm living proof. For instance, if I say I'm going to cut out dairy as a health goal, I work pretty diligently to make that happen. But occasionally I'll have some cheese or an egg, and I am okay with that—I've already cut out dairy 80 percent of the time. The ultimate point here is to forgive yourself for getting off track once in a while. Think of it this way: getting off track is actually part of the plan.

One of my goals, a few years back, was to cut down on my meat consumption and only consume meat once a week. This was part of my overall goal to ensure that 90 percent of the foods I consumed were plant-based and unprocessed or minimally processed foods. Were there weeks where I had meat or fish more than once a week? Of course! However, there were other weeks where I consumed zero meat or seafood. Prior to this commitment, I was eating meat every single day. The reality is that even if I 'cheat' every once in a while, I am still 80 percent better than before I committed to this change. Initially allowing myself to eliminate meat from my diet 80 percent of the time has now led to taking the meat out of my diet 100 percent of the time, and I actually cannot remember the last time I had any meat whatsoever.

THE BENEFITS OF A PLANT-BASED DIET

In order to optimize your health, I suggest you eat a diet mainly of plant-based, whole foods or minimally processed foods 80 percent of the time. This is the magic bullet. Nothing too sexy or exciting, is it? I wish it was a red or blue pill, and you only had to make a choice once.

Eating a whole-food, plant-based diet means having meals comprised mostly of non-processed foods, fruits, vegetables, nuts, and seeds. This is one of the reasons I start every single day with my 2-liter shake full of fruits and vegetables. By doing this, I get more than my required amount of fruits and vegetables and flood my system with healthy nutrients, minerals, and noninflammatory goodness.

Think of our ancestors, who worked their farms and ate non-processed foods like bread, milk, and eggs, fruits, and vegetables. When people ate this way and ate natural food from the land (think 'farm to table' when you shop), foods were fresher, more nutrient-dense and, therefore, the incidence of life-threatening illness and disease from diet was much, much lower.

Sticking to a plant-based diet shifts the focus from processed foods to whole foods. A reliance on processed foods also increases the risk of possibly introducing more chemicals, additional additives and other harmful agents into your body. For example, I've noticed how different bread and pasta are in North America versus Europe. A friend of mine can't eat any local bread, as he has a severe reaction to wheat and gluten (although he does not have celiac disease). He got violently ill whenever he consumed any processed bread products. Last year, he traveled to Italy and regularly consumed bread, pizza, and pasta with no reaction to the wheat or gluten whatsoever. This is possibly due to the different ways of processing foods (or not processing foods) in Europe, the use of pesticides, and differences in the use of non-hybridized wheat. While contrary to popular belief, wheat in North America is not technically genetically modified.

I bike race in Sardinia, Italy, and when I travel there, I consume a good amount of bread, pasta, and even baked goods with no reaction or upset stomach whatsoever, yet while at home, I tend to feel much more bloated and uncomfortable eating so much of these foods. In his book *Blue Zones*, author Dan Buettner (one of my favorite authors), gives readers insight into the habits and diets of the longest living people in the world, from Sardinia to Japan. In it, he outlines the habits of centenarians, and what struck me is the similarity of habits and routines of the longest living people on the planet.

Sardinia, Italy, happens to be one of the geographic areas with a large number of centenarians. I believe one of the reasons for this is the population's consumption of non-processed foods. The food that Sardinians eat is often fresh, organic, and farm to table.

Another one of my very favorite books on health and wellness is

How Not to Die, by Dr. Michael Greger. Dr. Greger shares the leading causes of death, including heart disease, diabetes, and stroke, and shares how to combat these, as well as many other diseases. As you read, you quickly realize that to combat all these diseases means looking hard at the foods we consume. From his years of research, Dr. Greger is a proponent of a whole food, plant-based diet, as it can reduce the risk of most illnesses and even reverse certain illnesses people may already have.

He cites a growing body of evidence that shows the health benefits of a vegetarian or vegan diet. A recent study from the Netherlands, for example, involved 6,000 people and found that those who ate a high ratio of plant protein compared to animal protein were at a lower risk of developing heart disease later in life. Another study from Brazil involving 4,500 subjects found that people who consumed a diet rich in plant protein were 60 percent less likely than their meat-eating counterparts to develop a buildup of plaque in the arteries of the heart.

Through my personal research, and input from Barb and our children as they began to go plant-based, as well as from my friend and mentor Rich Roll, I switched to a mainly plant-based diet. I didn't do it all at once—I listened to my own advice and took baby steps. But the results proved amazing. All my blood tests started routinely coming back with startling improvements and signaled my baseline health indicators were 'off the charts,' and not just in my own age bracket. This continues today. In addition, I have more energy, sleep better, and am able to have harder, better workouts than I did years ago. In fact, I've managed to qualify to represent Canada for the last five years in the World Triathlon Championships. I know this would not have been possible without changing my diet to mainly plant-based, non-processed foods.

I think Hippocrates had the right idea when he said, "Let food be thy medicine and medicine be thy food."

I encourage you to try a diet comprised mainly of plants, including fruits and vegetables, nuts and seeds and whole grains, and you will see changes in how you feel in a matter of days.

HOW TO BEGIN

But how to get started on this new course, this new relationship with food? A relationship you will have for the rest of your life? And when will this new approach to food feel natural and not precious or temporary? Well, I'm going to share with you some of my other daily rituals around eating. Take what works or sounds interesting to you and try it out, discard what doesn't. Try your own strategies. This should be a creative endeavor.

The first thing I do when I wake up, even before getting into shake-making mode, is go downstairs and prepare a cup of warm water with lemon or apple cider vinegar. There are several reasons for this. Some health practitioners believe the vitamin C in half a lemon has benefits, including that it may boost your immune system or help balance the pH balance in your body or curb hunger cravings. But even if that's not true, I feel hydrated at the start of my day when I begin with a tall glass of lemon water.

The benefits of apple cider vinegar are many. Hippocrates, for example, the father of modern medicine, used it to clean wounds and fight infection in the 4th century BCE.

Since then, cider vinegar has been used for everything from

fighting lice and warts to ear infections. Numerous studies have shown how apple cider vinegar can improve insulin function and help fight Type 2 diabetes. Other research shows that cider can increase satiety, lower cholesterol, and improve the overall health of your heart. I figure even if only half these benefits turn out to be real, it's worth trying to see if there are benefits for you. The key thing to remember is to take it in small doses, like 1 to 2 teaspoons in a cup of in a cup of warm, filtered water. More could potentially give you indigestion or affect the enamel on your teeth.

I also take vitamins with my Wilson Shake. I have an assortment of vitamins I take based on my blood work, which I have done two to three times a year and shows me any deficiencies I need to address. My vitamin choices change depending on my racing schedule. For example, I might take more vitamin C, curcumin, or turmeric, all of which are great for the immune system and reducing inflammation, depending upon what I'm training for. On a daily basis, I've stuck mostly to taking a good-quality multivitamin as well as vitamins B, C and D, plus magnesium supplements. Of course, before you adopt any regimen of vitamins, it's best to review it with your health-care provider.

DIETS DON'T WORK

We live in a world where we are constantly bombarded by information about what to eat and not eat, what the latest diet fad is that will shrink our waistline or increase our longevity. It's understandable that you might feel overwhelmed or confused about how to find a method of eating or dieting that is right for you.

Here's the thing: Diets don't work. They just don't. Study after study demonstrates how weight is often gained right back once the patient is off the diet. Diets are temporary and don't stick long term. Think of a diet for when you have four weeks to slim down enough to fit into your tux for your son's wedding, or maybe you want to sport a bikini for the first time in a few years on your Hawaiian vacation.

'Diet' shouldn't mean a temporary fix. From here on out, I will use the word diet in its broader sense, to refer to what you put in your mouth to sustain yourself.

Ah. Feel better? You should. Think of it as fine-tuning your eating habits in line with a permanent lifestyle change and not a diet.

Changing your eating habits to fit a lifestyle change means you are really buckling down and trying to create more good habits than bad regarding what you put in your body. There are so many choices when it comes to eating lifestyles, from paleo to keto, raw food vegan to vegetarian. Not every diet works for every person or is sustainable over time. I chose a primarily plant-based, or vegan, diet that works for me. A couple of things worth noting, though: All of these seemingly disparate eating styles avoid processed foods of any kind, and are devoid of high fructose corn syrup as well as hydrogenated oils. Sometimes what you're *not* eating is just as important as what you are.

Barb and I have three kids, all in their 20s, and they are all very physically active. They've always played a lot of sports, and a couple of them have played football in college and competed at the national level in Canada in both skiing and CrossFit. My daughter and my eldest son are 100 percent vegan, and my younger son, the one who made the national team for ski cross and is now trying to qualify for the World CrossFit Games, eats some grass-fed and organic meat, consuming only very 'clean' food. I am mostly vegan, but I do eat some fish. Barb and I started this nutritional journey together, which definitely makes it easier than if you are the odd person out in your household and trying to eat clean.

Again, I can't overstate the fact that my family has always been active and athletic, and I certainly used to believe that physical activity was the only thing I needed to pay attention to in order to maintain my health. As I wrote earlier, when the kids were little it was a family ritual to stop at Dairy Queen after whatever game we'd attended and have a honking big ice cream sundae. As a parent of young kids, I was running and going to the gym, but I wasn't focused on eating as a way of being healthy. I just want you to understand that how I got where I am today has been a slow evolution and not something that happened overnight. Eventually, whatever plan you decide to adopt, it needs to be sustainable—that is, something you will consistently do over a lifetime.

This should help you see that I did not start out going full-on vegan. If I had, it probably wouldn't have stuck as a lifestyle for me. I've found I feel my best when I eat this way. But it happened gradually—I went from eating red meat four or five times a week to only treating myself to it on the weekend. A steak dinner and a glass of wine remained in my diet but only on Saturday nights. Slowly, however, even meat disappeared from my plate. But I never woke up one day and said, "Today I'm vegan." I deviated from time to time, like maybe on a special holiday or family celebration, or if my son was going to have a steak, I'd have one with him. But as of this writing, I can't even remember the last time I had red meat.

HOW I EAT

If you're wondering what a daily vegan menu might look like, I do eat a lot of salads. But they're not always your typical green salads. For example, at lunch, a salad for me may include different types of lettuce like a spring mix, plus cucumbers, peppers, carrots and onions. For dinner, I might combine rice, quinoa, seeds, vegetables, and sweet potatoes in a bowl and then finish it off with some arugula and hot sauce—and it's delicious and easy! I've included recipes at the back of the book to get you started, but they're meant to be a guide only. Meal prep is really about trial and error, using what you have, and tailoring foods to your taste buds.

Sometimes, you do find yourself in a situation where you don't have a lot of choices about what to eat. Maybe you're at a buffet-style dinner or even a plated dinner for a work event, and what's being served is not the healthiest. I never want to be that guy who makes a big fuss about what I have to eat. So, I'm more likely to take a bite or two of whatever's on offer and just not eat the rest. Again, just channel the 80/20 Rule. Unless you have a food allergy, you have an intolerance to gluten or have celiac disease, then you can most likely eat a bit of something not on your usual lifestyle eating plan. And that's fine—enjoy nibbling and then come home to your own healthy meal.

I used to drink milk every day. Then my kids started giving me a hard time. How could I adopt a plant-based diet when I drink milk? In their eyes, I couldn't call myself plant-based if I drank milk. But they had a point; milk doesn't make the grade when eating plant-based. Gradually, I switched to almond or cashew milk in my coffee, then eventually, I got used to just having coffee black. As with everything in this chapter, the focus is on baby steps. Rome wasn't built in a day. Your eating habits don't change overnight. Change what you can, eliminate the worst offenders, start eating whole, unprocessed foods, and you're already halfway there.

These steps are easy, attainable, inexpensive, and you can do them immediately.

I first gravitated toward a vegan diet because of the health benefits it offers. But as the years have passed, I find myself preferring this way of eating for more philosophical and ethical reasons. I believe it is more sustainable for the planet and simply more humane. Though there has been a rise in awareness of sustainable and organic farming methods for raising and slaughtering livestock, there are still far too many factory farms that treat animals inhumanely and, further, create extraordinary levels of greenhouse gas emissions for our already stretched planet reeling with the challenges of climate change.

I used to fish a lot at our cottage in Muskoka, Ontario. I would catch the fish, clean them, and cook them. Last year, my son Matt wanted to eat fish for his birthday. We went out to the lake and caught some fish. But as we were cleaning them, both of us realized we were feeling pretty bad about it. Both of us felt guilty about taking the fish's life for our dinner. I know it sounds crazy, but this is just how my awareness and thinking have changed. It's not for everybody, and I don't judge anyone who eats meat. For me, over time, it has become an unsustainable choice. That's the key: over time.

MORE RESOURCES

I cannot close this chapter without mentioning a book that has had a huge influence on me: *The China Study* by T. Colin Campbell. This comprehensive book examines the link between eating meat and various forms of chronic illnesses and cancers. The exhaustive research detailed in the book concludes that a diet based on whole foods and plants, without any animal products, is the healthiest eating plan. It's based on a 20-year study conducted by the Chinese Academy of Preventive Medicine, Cornell University, and the University of Oxford. I have never needed more evidence than what's in this book that a vegan diet is the healthiest option. But what works for me doesn't necessarily work for another person, and you will need to draw your own conclusions.

Another highly useful and inspirational resource is the work of Dr. Valter Longo, the director of the University of Southern California's Longevity Institute in Los Angeles. Dr. Longo is one of the world's leading experts on fasting—and every form it can take. His book *The Longevity Diet: Discover the New Science Behind Stem Cell Activation and Regeneration to Slow Aging, Fight Disease, and Optimize Weight*, brings together the benefits of fasting with a diet plan that mimics its effects to keep your system in optimal shape and add years to your life.

According to Longo's work, high-protein diets such as Paleo and Atkins are the least healthy option for people. Growth hormones in humans are powerful metabolic chemicals that stimulate the growth of almost all body tissues and enhance lean body mass. Pathways in cells, including TOR and IGF-1, are controlled by proteins, and they are accelerators of the aging process. The evidence suggests that if you eat a low-protein diet, you may live longer and healthier.

I had considered Longo's research on fasting and now integrate some form of intermittent fasting into my daily routine, limiting the hours I eat in the day. One of the toughest things our body has to do each day is digest the different foods we consume. I've found that by limiting my food intake to a 12-hour period over the day really helps my energy level the next day. I find that when I have my last meal of the day between 6 and 7 p.m., and don't eat again until the next morning at 7 or 8 a.m., my energy level and my mental acuity are significantly better. Some days, I even extend this fasting window until lunch, which means I extend my fasting period to 16 hours. When the human body doesn't have to expend this energy on digesting food, our body has energy for other necessary functioning. I like to periodically give myself a fasting period of 13 to 16 hours.

CHECKLIST: EATING WELL

Improve your eating habits by following these steps:

- Get your blood work done to find out where you might be deficient in vitamins and minerals, and to determine if you have elevated cholesterol, blood pressure or sugar levels.
- Keep a food diary for a week to find out what you're really ingesting. If 'diary' sounds too complicated, just make notes on The Wheels of Health Daily Log on page 174, or your phone or calendar.
- Try making The Wilson Shake (see the Recipes section on page 126). Now do it again but make your own version. Try doing it three out of seven mornings. If you like it, commit to five days and see how that feels.
- Drink warm lemon water or warm water with a shot of apple cider vinegar first thing in the morning before your coffee or tea. Notice if this helps your digestion and keeps you hydrated.
- Try to shift your diet to mainly whole foods, mainly plant-based and non-processed.
- Keep the 80/20 Rule in mind—if you mess up, don't sweat it! Take baby steps toward better food choices. That's the path to long-term success.
- Try intermittent fasting, where you don't consume any food or drink (other than water) from dinnertime until the next morning.

WHEEL 2:

Exercise

My daughter, Lauren, and I were staying at Whistler Mountain, located in the Garibaldi Provincial Park in British Columbia. In winter, Whistler is a skier's paradise; in summer, it belongs to hikers, mountain bikers, rock climbers and other outdoor enthusiasts. It is one of the nicest places in the world. We try to go, with various members of our family, for a few weeks every summer.

This particular week in August was part of what we called Training Week. We did massive hikes, bike rides, or runs every day. My family supports what I would say is a mostly healthy and spirited level of competition among the five of us, who are all sporty and physically active. My kids will never shy away from the challenge of trying to beat me in any competition, and I return the favor. Therefore, it will be no surprise that by the end of the week, Lauren and I had decided we were going to run up Whistler Mountain together. I wasn't entirely sure if we were running up together or to see who landed at the top first. But seriously, the main point was we were doing it together.

To give you an idea of the task at hand, Whistler Mountain is almost 7,500 feet high, and it is a 27-kilometer run up as you wind up to the peak. It might not be Mount Everest, but it's still a challenge. By the time our last day rolled around, we were both exhausted. Lauren said to me, "I don't think we're going to do it."

All week I had been the one who didn't want to do it. Well, that changed.

"No, no," I replied. I had all our stuff ready to go. "We *are* going to do it."

Lauren agreed, and we set out running up the mountain—all 27 kilometers of it. Slowly, mind you, and every half hour, we'd stop for 30 seconds and switch who was carrying the backpack, which contained some vegan energy bars and water. We ran that way for 4½ hours up to Whistler's summit.

We both felt it was an achievement that needed to be memorialized in some way. Standing on the top of the mountain and looking around for miles at the stunning panorama, I said, "We're going to make a commitment right now. We're going to run up the mountain every year for the next 25 years from now on [until I'm 80 years old]. I can't promise I'm going to run all the way, but I'll try. And if not, we'll hike up."

She put out her hand and shook mine. "It's a date, Dad." We wrote the promise in our logbook, where we note all our hikes. As I write this book, we are planning our run up the mountain for the third time.

As you can see, I'm interested in longevity and staying active. I figure the best chance I have of making that happen for me is to plan for it. Research referenced in the book *Blue Zones* shows that among the centenarians studied, one of the common factors contributing to their long lives was that they move their bodies and stay active. In North America, and probably most of the Westernized world, I think we spend far too much time in our cars and sitting at desks all day.

MORNING ROUTINES

If you make a conscious effort to start every day with some kind of movement, that can set you on the right path to staying active for much longer. Here are some morning rituals I've put in place for myself that start my day off on the right foot. (All puns intended.)

When I wake up early in the morning, the first thing I do is open my curtains and let in the light, whatever there is of it. I want the daylight to hit my eyes right away, so it helps me wake up. Some people bound out of bed in the morning, but I am more likely to give myself a few minutes to meditate or gather my thoughts before getting up and fixing myself a cup of warm water with lemon or apple cider vinegar. After that, I head down to my basement and hop on my bike trainer, do a weight workout, or head out the door for a ride, a swim, or a run.

My workouts vary from day to day, but I find if I get my workout done first thing in the morning, it gets my circulation and energy up right away. I may go for 45 minutes to an hour or more, depending upon my schedule. I'll often do a workout in the gym later in the day with weights, but in the morning, it's almost always cardio. If I'm training for a triathlon race, I'll run, cycle or swim every day, mixing it up to keep me interested and my body in shape. Though I have a makeshift gym in my basement, I also go to the YMCA if I have a swim workout scheduled or when I have more time on the weekends. On really busy days, when the gym is out of the question, I just try to do something involving moving, like a walk or a hike or even yoga.

After my workout I'll have a shower, and for the last five minutes I stand under freezing cold water.

There are numerous benefits to a cold shower at the end of your hot one, which might seem counterintuitive at first. Of course, athletes have long used ice baths after training to soothe sore muscles. The benefits of a cold shower work in much the same way.

Cold showers can boost both your immune system and your metabolism, enabling you to burn more fat during the day. They also make you more alert and leave you feeling invigorated, rather than drowsy from the usual dose of hot water. There are even benefits to your skin and hair from cold water. Hot water can dry out your skin much faster, as it can strip hair and skin of healthy oils. The cold water can even make your hair appear shinier and healthier by flattening the hair follicles.

The age-old practice of swimming in cold water in the winter, as exemplified by the Canadian Polar Bear plunges on New Year's Day, supports long-held folk wisdom on the benefits of cold water. A study from Humboldt University in Berlin, Germany, first found a decrease in the uric acid levels of regular winter swimmers. This finding was replicated in many other experiments, including a recent one that showed how cold-water therapy can decrease cell damage after exercise. The exposure to cold increases the body's production of glutathione, a naturally occurring antioxidant in the body, which helps all the other elements in your body's metabolism function optimally.

Finally, it will give your mood a boost. You will be hopping out of that cold shower with far more energy and vitality than you stepped into it. Believe me.

There are definitely some days when I don't have time for a morning workout. In that case, I'll do 20 push-ups or do some stretching to get my body moving and my heart rate going a bit before hopping in the shower. Sometimes I also stand and bounce in one spot or run up and down the stairs a few times. Anything I can do to get my body moving. For some people, it might be doing a few minutes of yoga to wake up the body, stretch, and increase flexibility. But I do encourage you to try something you like first thing in the morning or when you first wake.

CHANGE YOUR EXPECTATIONS ABOUT AGING

Building a morning ritual around moving—even just a baby step at a time—helps to put in place a foundation for getting into healthy habits that will increase both your health and longevity. A lot of people have an expectation that "I'm 60, 65, or 70, so I'm going to slow down." I'm almost 60 now, and it's not a big thing for me to run for an hour or cycle for 2 hours or more. That may sound very impressive, but believe me, when you work up to it as I have, it's not that hard to do. There are thousands of people out there 10 years older than me who routinely run marathons. The internal shift I'm encouraging you to make is in the ability to change your expectations about not only what you think you deserve, but also what you think you're capable of.

I'm not saying it's not difficult to change your old ways of thinking, but I'm living proof that it can be done. I am not superhuman, but I've learned the people you surround yourself with will have a big impact on your success. Just like in other areas of your life, those around you influence you. Living a healthy lifestyle is no different. Think of this more as a shift in your mindset, rather than some massive change.

If you sit around thinking about how your body is falling apart and nothing can be done... well, nothing will be done. But if you surround yourself with people who are perhaps older than you, physically active, and enjoying their physical activities, your frame of reference shifts. Being active becomes the new normal.

According to the Mayo Clinic, there is a clear and discernible link between the effect of exercise and mood. The release of endorphins into your bloodstream literally lifts your spirit. So, while it's understandable that maybe the last thing you feel like doing is exercising if you're depressed or going through a major life change like a divorce, death of a loved one, or job change, it might just be the very thing that tips the scales toward an improved outlook and feeling of well-being.

MAKE EXERCISE JOYFUL

I have been fortunate that I've always been able to work out with my family. And by 'with' I mean sometimes with various members strapped to me. When my kids were little, we scheduled workouts around their activities and took them to the nursery at the gym. I was that guy you see running while pushing the buggy as the kid squeals with delight, the wind in his hair. I don't think it's an accident my kids have wound up being very active people, too. They've been around exercise and steeped in the joy of physical activity their whole lives.

Whenever possible, I always choose to exercise outdoors rather than staying inside the gym. There is something far more invigorating about exercising outside and being close to nature than sweating in a large room filled with other damp people, often with loud music not of your choosing. Studies demonstrate how moving your body helps not only with depression and mental illness but also offers an added benefit from being undertaken outdoors. How can you pass up that two-for-one deal?

We have a natural, evolved affinity with nature, what biologist E. O. Wilson called 'biophilia.' One of his well-known studies found that people who were hospitalized recovered much quicker when they had a view of trees and clouds or flowers out their window instead of a brick wall.

The field of environmental psychology found the three biggest benefits we get from spending time in nature are a reduction in stress levels, improvement in mood, and improvement in cognitive performance. In addition, science is finding that it's not just psychological benefits we derive from being in nature; there may also be a bacterium that leads to a higher resistance to stress. It's called

Mycobacterium vaccae and has been found to induce the release of the serotonin, which acts as a neurotransmitter, in the brains of mice. Serotonin, also known as the happy chemical, is associated with stabilizing mood among many other functions, including regulating appetite, sleep, and memory.

GET STARTED

The body responds to exercise almost immediately, and that's good news to keep you motivated. If you need to take baby steps, then do it. Walk half a mile every day for three days. Then rest. On the fifth day, you will double the distance to a mile.

> **Your body wants to be fit. It evolved to run and lift and jump and climb. The moment you begin investing time in physical activity, the better you will feel. Immediately.**

The idea of a connection between the mind and body is built on a false construct. It's not about connecting two separate entities. It is all one elaborate, complicated machine. What we feed the engine, i.e., how we treat the body, impacts the brain and cognition, it can put off or eliminate the threat of dementia. Circulation of both blood and lymph fluids keeps the body and immune system fit and the brain functioning at its best.

Whatever you're doing, when you're tired, or you think you can't get out of bed and run, consider this: What if it wasn't a choice? What if you couldn't run? What if you couldn't turn your head to change lanes, or bring in a bag of groceries? The worst thing isn't doing the exercise. The worst thing is not being able to do it.

Find something you like to do and go do it. It doesn't matter what it is.

CHECKLIST: EXERCISE

Step up your physical activity by adding these actions to your daily routine:

- Do something to get your body moving and blood circulating first thing in the morning. It doesn't matter what it is—just move. This could be a walk, cycle, yoga, stretching, jumping jacks, push-ups, or full-on workout.
- Finish your normal shower with a cold burst of water for one to two minutes or as long as you can stand it. You will be invigorated and have supercharged your metabolism and immune system for the day.
- Incorporate movement into your day as much as possible. Take the stairs instead of the elevator. Make a game out of counting your steps for the day, either with a health app on your smartphone, fitness tracker like a Fitbit, or a pedometer. If you're getting in anywhere from 5,000 to 10,000 steps a day, you're golden.
- Involve other members of your family or your friends in your moving activities. If you can find an exercise or accountability buddy you're more likely to accomplish your movement goals.
- Get outdoors and in nature as much as possible. This will elevate your mood and decrease stress levels.
- Track what you do. If you don't have an exercise routine, try for three days a week. Then bump it up to four. See The Wheels of Health Daily Log on page 172 for a template to record your routine.
- Incorporate cardio activities like walking, running, or cycling, as well as resistance training (weights or bands) into your weekly routine.

Sleep

Trying to get a good night's sleep can be a lot like herding cats. Sleeping disorders are one of the top 10 complaints people take to their doctors. The lack of adequate sleep is a chronic problem for 39 percent of North Americans. So much has been written about this 'sleep epidemic,' as it has been referred to in the media, that I'm sure none of this will come as much of a surprise.

The Public Health Agency of Canada reports that one in three adults aged 35 to 64 are not getting enough sleep, and half of all adults have trouble going to sleep or staying asleep. Another one in three say they have difficulty staying awake during waking hours.

Clearly, lack of sleep is a problem. The fact many people don't get enough of it can be due to numerous factors like stress, 24/7 on-demand media, shift work, or simply stimulants like caffeine, nicotine, and alcohol. People have trouble getting to sleep, staying asleep, and sleeping at the appropriate time. When you start falling asleep during your meetings, you can be sure you're not getting enough uninterrupted sleep at night.

ADOPTING GOOD SLEEP RITUALS

One thing you can do to help yourself is to adopt good sleep rituals. Your body takes cues from your habits. If you start doing the same things before bedtime every night at roughly the same time, your body will learn that's the time for sleep. Sleep is triggered by a potent cocktail of hormones, a lack of light, and the biological need to repair.

Like you, I always have things on my mind. In the past, sometimes I'd sleep like a baby, while other nights I'd wake up at 3 a.m. and not get back to sleep. The second I'd open my eyes, even in the middle of the night, I'd be thinking of something. In order to quiet my mind as much as possible, I created a routine I do every night, starting an hour before bed. These rituals worked and now, with rare exceptions, I sleep a full night without waking up.

SETTING UP A SLEEP ENVIRONMENT

I try to shut off all electronics and devices at least an hour before bed. If I'm going to read on my tablet, I'll make sure it's set to nighttime reading, which knocks out the blue light that keeps the brain activated. I actually do this with all my devices—set them to automatically block out the sleep-inhibiting blue light at a set time. I also make sure my room is very dark and cool.

SUPPLEMENTING MY SLEEP

I ensure I'm getting plenty of magnesium in my diet. I usually take a magnesium supplement, so I know I'm consuming enough of this essential macronutrient. The body doesn't produce magnesium on its own and must find it in outside sources, such as dark leafy vegetables, seeds, and nuts, squash, broccoli, legumes, dairy, meat, unprocessed grains, chocolate, and coffee. You can see why I take the supplements, as I don't eat dairy or meat.

Magnesium also helps control your body's stress response system, and it increases gamma-aminobutyric acid (GABA) in the body, which helps with relaxation necessary for sleep. I take magnesium glycinate and magnesium malate right before I go to bed, and the effect is real. My system relaxes, and sleep follows almost immediately.

I also take ZMA, which is a zinc and magnesium supplement that promotes sleep. The zinc helps your body absorb the magnesium into your system. I also drink an herbal tea—a chamomile mix—which leaves me feeling calm.

EXPRESSING GRATITUDE

I do this every night before I go to sleep. Once I turn out the light, I go into what I call my positive focus, something I adopted from one of my mentors, Dan Sullivan, but you could equally call it a gratitude checklist. I think of three things that I'm grateful for during that particular day. It could be something as simple as a call with my children, or a hike I went on with my wife, or maybe I had a great sales meeting. Some days are tougher than others, and it can be hard to think of three things, but it can be kept very simple. It's just good practice to get into framing issues and incidences in a positive light, no matter what they are. After that, I'm usually able to drift off to sleep.

ADDING MEDITATION TO THE MIX

Of course, things don't go according to plan every night. There are times when I have a whole lot on my mind, and I still wake at 3 o'clock and can't get back to sleep. A few years ago, I went through a period of 3 a.m. wake-ups, and when that happened I took to getting up and going for a run.

I do not recommend this approach to deal with chronic insomnia, as I would end up more tired the next day from my nocturnal workout. It can become a vicious cycle; being more tired during the day, and when night comes, more stressed about being able to sleep, which then leads to more insomnia. It's counterintuitive, and if you haven't been through it you might be hard-pressed to believe that if you're extremely tired you could have trouble sleeping, but it happens. You can get yourself into a wired and anxious state about not sleeping, and that is the last thing you need.

After a few of my nighttime runs, I went to discuss my insomnia with my doctor. He put a monitor on my finger to measure brain activity and asked me, "How stressed are you on a scale of one to 10?"

I said, "I don't know, maybe four or five."

He turned the screen around to show me, and it was bright red—off the charts.

"That's the activity that's going on in your brain right now. Your brain activity is just going crazy. Have you ever meditated?" he asked.

I admitted I hadn't, well aware that wasn't the answer he wanted.

"Let me take you through a five-minute meditation session," he said. I then had an intimate introduction to my own breathing. We just focused on the breath. He turned the screen around again, and literally, within a minute of starting that meditation session, the screen flashed to green. This meant I had completely calmed my brain activity. Red to green, just like that.

Before this exercise, however, I didn't even know my brain was overly active or that I could calm it.

What this showed me was the importance of just slowing down, even for five minutes a day. This is how I first began implementing meditation in my life, and it made a huge difference in being able to relax at night, fall asleep, and even get back to sleep if I woke up.

Meditation and conscious breathing is the last tool I use to set the stage for a solid seven to nine hours of sleep. (See Deep Breathing Exercise, page 73.)

My sleep rituals extend to when I wake up in the morning. You read earlier how I open my drapes first thing, and here's one big reason why I do it. I know it's important to get my eyes fixed on whatever sunlight there is to help my body naturally release melatonin and kick-start my day. Exposure to light in the morning, when it has the biggest impact, then ramps up the production of serotonin, which is converted to melatonin to help us sleep much later that night. With the sun's rays streaming in, I relax in bed for a few minutes before getting up for the day and think about what's in store over the next 12 hours. Then I rise, knowing I've rested both body and mind and am in the best shape to meet the day.

THE SCIENCE OF SLEEP

Sleep studies have come a long way in the last decade. Everyone's sleep needs are different and are often predictable by age. Most adults need at least seven to nine hours of sleep, and yet 80 percent of adults 25 to 60 claim to get between four and six hours a night. This kind of chronic sleep deprivation can potentially lead to dementia, Parkinson's disease, brain fog, and, most certainly, physical exhaustion. The brain has no lymph nodes, which means there's no way for the body to clean the brain. Instead, the brain shrinks at night, by up to one-third, allowing synovial fluid to essentially 'wash' the brain and allow toxins like free radicals and plaque-producing enzymes to be filtered through the liver. An hour before you wake, your blood pressure rises, your brain returns to its full size, and hormones prepare your body to rise and face the day.

In his book *The Sleep Solution*, author M. Chris Winter, M.D., talks about his theory of primary drives. We all have a primary drive for food, water, sleep, and sex (and not in any particular order!), he states. So even if we feel we don't sleep or don't sleep enough or well, we still sleep, and the body gets what it needs. Basically, the brain will do anything eventually, when push comes to shove, to get your body to sleep.

Even if you feel you struggle with insomnia, the first step is to accept that you do actually sleep. From there, you can work on how to get more and better sleep.

One of the most tried and true methods to address insomnia, according to Dr. Winter and other practitioners of sleep wisdom, is to use a form of cognitive behavioral therapy (CBT) for fixing your sleep problems. This involves limiting the time you spend in bed when you are not sleeping, so you come to associate your bed only with sleep (and sex) but nothing else. You start by picking a wake-up time that will remain consistent every morning. For example, if you pick 7 in the morning, you'd take the last amount of sleep you think you got, say four hours. Your new bedtime for the next few nights will be 3 in the morning. Yes, you read that right. You're training your brain and body to associate bed with sleeping, not with lying awake.

Once you're getting into bed and sleeping a solid four hours, you move your bedtime back between 15 minutes and half an hour every night, until you're getting the amount of sleep that leaves you feeling refreshed and functional the next day. The lasting key to success here, according to Dr. Winter, is to set both your bedtime and wake up time the same every day and to absolutely never waver from them.

The other critically important thing is to notice how you talk about sleep and how you react when you're having trouble sleeping. Instead of complaining about how tired you are, try skipping that step and focusing on something positive instead. Compliment someone on their new shoes instead of complaining about how you slept like crap the night before. I don't mean to get all woo-woo on you, but I believe it's just a law of nature that the more you put negative energy toward something, the more you give that thing power in your life.

To that same end, if you're lying in bed getting frustrated because you're not falling asleep for the first time or settling back to sleep at 4 a.m., try distracting yourself by reading a mindless book, or maybe getting up for a few minutes and doing some simple tasks around the house that don't involve any brainpower. I often go downstairs, keep the lights dimmed and make myself an herbal calming tea. It can sometimes be just enough to make you feel like you're at least getting something useful done while you're having trouble falling asleep. Whatever the activity is will depend on you and your own circumstances, but anything is better than trying to chase that elusive sleep.

The bottom line is don't shortchange yourself on sleep if at all possible.

CHECKLIST: SLEEP

Get more zzzs and a better quality sleep with these tips:

- Prioritize sleep in your life. It's the glue that holds everything together. Without it, you compromise the other spokes of your wheel.
- Try going to sleep an hour earlier than usual. This is the number one thing I did to improve my sleep.
- Adopt a sleep ritual that works for you. For example, a certain kind of relaxing music you listen to before bed, a warm bath, meditation, yoga, or reading.
- Make sure your room is as dark, quiet, and as cool as possible. If the steady sound of something helps you fall asleep, use a white noise machine or fan.
- Refrain from using electronics, phones, or computers at least two hours before bed.
- Avoid eating a heavy meal too late at night and keep alcohol

and nicotine to a minimum two to three hours before bed. (Or, better yet, avoid them altogether).

- Don't drink caffeine after 3 o'clock in the afternoon.
- Do a gratitude check just before you go to sleep. Think of three simple things that happened that day that you're grateful for, even if it's just that the sun was shining.
- Incorporate meditation into your daily routine as a means to get to sleep and quiet the chatter in your head. There are many meditation apps today, and most are free. Try a lesson a day for three or four days and then try one at night. Keep practicing! More on this later in the book.
- Add a deep breathing exercise to your bedtime routine (see exercise below).

BONUS: DEEP BREATHING EXERCISE

I find the practice of deep breathing much easier than meditation, and studies have shown that even five deep, slow breaths have an impact on slowing your body and your mind. The methods I use most often are:

- Box Breathing: Breathe in, hold, and breathe out for the same number of seconds when breathing in. Do it 10 times. So for example, I will do five seconds in, five seconds hold and five seconds breathing out, and repeat the pattern 10 times.
- 4, 7, 8 Breathing: Breathe in for four seconds, hold for seven, exhale for eight. This serves to activate your parasympathetic nervous system, which is your 'relaxing' system that wards off stress.

I do these often throughout my day, as I find that when things get stressful, it's a great way to slow down your system and relax. I also breathe intentionally most nights in bed as a way to relax the system prior to falling asleep. Many nights I fall asleep before I even finish the deep breathing exercises!

Mindfulness

When my children and I are not setting ridiculous, competitive challenges for ourselves, we can often be found taking a more meditative Zone Two run through the woods near our house or cottage. Zone Two refers to the level of effort; you're not doing a heavy cardio workout but more of a fast walk or easy meditative run or ride. The whole idea of the Zone Two run is to put easy stress on the system, and try to be in the present moment as much as possible.

Try to really perceive what's going on around you. Look at the birds, the trees, the flowers, and just try to focus on the present moment and your breath. This is truly a form of meditation. We always think that in order to meditate, we have to be sitting on a cushion with our back pillar straight and our eyes closed. But being mindful means just that: being aware of your surroundings and focusing on the input without allowing thoughts to intrude. This is really the meaning of being mindful, and you can reap great benefits from it in the form of stress-reduction and peace of mind.

I have a series of mantras—thoughts I use to help me focus my meditation—I say every time I go running or for a walk, which help me stay focused on the present and be mindful of my surroundings. I find these offer real peace of mind and enable me to focus on what is happening right now.

I hear the birds that are a mile away, the drone of an airplane, the sound of wind blowing through the trees—all sounds I normally wouldn't even pay attention to. Here is a summary of some of the mantras I practiced while out for a recent run with Lauren. I use some of them when I exercise outdoors and others before going to sleep:

Mantra 1:
I Will Be Present

I notice everything that I am personally experiencing at that point in time. I listen to nature, the sounds of insects, and of birds chirping. I feel the wind on my face, notice the beauty all around me, hear my footsteps, the way I'm breathing, just to name a few. I become 100 percent present with my body, my surroundings, and all that is happening around me.

I focus on every step and every sensation, beginning with the breath. As I run, I become aware of every new piece of sensory information and simply note it. If thoughts of work or the week's problems begin to materialize and intrude, I note them, too, and then let those thoughts go. I tell myself that dedicating time to run or walk, free of all those things-I-gotta-do, is a worthwhile endeavour. I pay attention to what I'm seeing, hearing, and experiencing now, in the present.

Mantra 2:
I Am Grateful for My Life

There is more and more being written about the power of the feeling of gratitude. In the book 13 *Things Mentally Strong People Don't Do*, author Amy Morin writes about the understated power of gratitude. When it costs nothing and is so easy to cultivate, it's a wonder more people don't know about this simple transformative life practice. According to a 2015 study published in the journal *Emotion*, acknowledging people's contributions and thanking people can lead to unexpected opportunities. Practicing gratitude also improves your health. A 2012 study in the journal *Personality and Individual Differences* discovered that people who regularly expressed gratitude experienced fewer aches and pains and were more likely to exercise often and attend regular wellness exams. Further studies have shown that gratitude also improves psychological health, reduces aggression, and improves mental strength. Finally, it's even been shown that people who jot down a few things they are grateful for before going to bed at night sleep better. With so much compelling evidence in favor of practicing gratitude, I'm hard-pressed to offer any downside to this mental and spiritual practice.

In case you're thinking all this gratitude research is conveniently drawn from people who are already happy, another recent study from the University of California, Berkeley set out to study 300 college students who were already seeking help for mental health issues like anxiety and depression. One group was asked to write a gratitude letter to someone for something they had done. Researchers followed up with them at four weeks and again at 12 weeks, and on both occasions, the group showed significantly better mental health than when they started the study. It was also found that a lack of negative words in the students' letters correlated with the reports of improved mental health at the four-week and 12-week marks.

Writing positively about someone else and reliving the gratitude, understanding gratitude fully, and defining it in their own terms increased the mental health of the participants.

I practice gratitude either during one of my runs through the woods or at the end of the day when I'm winding down. Wherever I am, after I've become aware of the physical world around me, I switch to focusing on what I am grateful for. During my run, I think deeply and profoundly of how much I appreciate my life, living and enjoying all life has to offer, and my family. Sometimes I conjure a kind of existential gratitude, where I feel aware of all the beauty in the world and what a miracle it is to be simply alive. At other times, I am grateful just to be able to bend over and put on my shoes and step out for a run.

I pay attention to the things that surround me and try to appreciate the small things in life. On a recent flight to the Giro Sardinia cycling race in the Mediterranean, the sun was setting over Toronto as we were taking off. I was taken aback by the beauty of the sun, the reflection of the sun on the plane's wings, and the urban, steely beauty of Toronto. As the flight progressed, I saw dawn. Flying over Europe, I allowed myself to be overwhelmed by the beauty and the miracle of a sunrise.

CELEBRATING BIG LITTLE THINGS

Recently I read an Instagram post celebrating the Big Little Things. When I first read that, it took me a moment to understand what it meant. It's all about those big moments when you are nourished by something you've noticed with intention, but that often go unseen by others because they are little things. It may be the laughter of your spouse, your partner, your children, the green of the blades of grass, the rays of sunlight shining through a window, falling snowflakes, the mist on a mirror after a hot shower, a home-cooked meal. The rainbows your eyelashes make when in direct sunlight. The list is endless.

I think there's a misconception that if we seek out the Big Things in life, those things are the only places we'll find happiness. For example, we go on trips, to lakes, to the mountains, to beaches, to Niagara Falls, to the CN Tower, all in a quest to find beauty and see those really 'Big' things. Don't get me wrong—those are all amazing places to visit, but my point is there are so many things around us every day that we generally don't notice or appreciate.

That kind of appreciation takes a certain amount of self-awareness and mindfulness. The way to help find the resources for learning how to be this aware, this mindful, is through meditation.

Meditation is a form of exercising your mind. Meditation is not passive. It is active. You are actively looking at the workings of your own mind and learning how to calm your brain.

If you try mediation just a few minutes a day, you will be further along on your journey than if you never tried it. There are endless studies demonstrating how meditating just 15 minutes a day lowers blood pressure, can help relieve mental distress and depression, is useful in anger management, and reduces recidivism in prison populations. Being aware of how your mind works and clearing that space for reflection is worth it.

Life is so busy, you may ask yourself, "How do I notice all the Big Little Things around me?" as that recent Instagram post urged.

Just take a minute before you react. Notice the person speaking to you. See them. When you're pumping gas, watch the sky for geese overhead, and look at the sunset. Really look. When you can't find your keys and are storming around the house, ask yourself, "How long do I want to be angry about this?" We often think we need to go on a hike, go to the mountains, or go to a lake to really appreciate all the world has to offer. The reality is, moments of pure clarity and beauty are all around us every single day—but you have to make an effort to isolate them, receive them, and make them happen for yourself.

SET ASIDE TIME TO SLOW DOWN AND TAKE NOTICE

I find that a great way to get in the habit of noticing these Big Little Things is to set aside time to slow down and take notice. I try to make a habit of going outside once a day and actively noticing all that is going on. In the spring, for example, the beauty all around is easy to see. The flights of birds, the sounds of their songs, the smell of the earth, the tumble of flowers, the warmth of the sun, or even the muggy properties of rain. When I can, I also try to enjoy my morning shake outside, close to nature, with the sun shining. This allows me to witness the day beginning to unfold. A day that will never repeat itself. Another day I am lucky enough to love others and be loved. Another day to be alive.

At night, before bed, I do the same thing. I generally go out back, and I look up and gaze at the stars, the moon, the reflection of moonlight against clouds, and planes flying overhead. In winter, the crisp smell of ice and snow is electrifying. In summer, the feel of the warm breeze and the wet smell of cut grass is moving. Once again, I am taking time out to appreciate all that is around me and how beautiful the world is, and it only takes a minute to perceive. Learning to frame your experiences is the key—that dense fog that forces an important meeting to be canceled also leaves your skin wet, makes your children's hair delightfully curly and is maybe weighted with the scent of roses from some neighbor's yard.

I have found that I no longer need to 'schedule' time to notice the beauty all around, as now I observe it naturally as I go through my day. So, you may ask, what can you do in order to notice the Big Little Things? It's quite simple. Take time today when you're driving, walking, or sitting outside, and spot all that surrounds you. Take note of the sky, the stars, the sun, the grass, the plants, the rain, the birds, etc. Take a different route to work. Notice the differences. Notice how this makes you feel. It is amazing how focusing on the details frees the mind.

Mantra 3:

I Celebrate All the Love in My Life

I think of Barb, our amazing children, my family, friends, and other people who have touched my life. I reflect on those who are no longer with us. This would include my mom and dad (Joanie and Howie), our grandparents and other family members that are no longer with us, to name a few. But I don't just think of their names. I work to remember a smile, how my mom was always so comforting, how my dad always had a grin on his face and was always there for me. To have known and loved them is a privilege. Having a near-death experience taught me that love is at once transforming and never-ending. If you focus on this idea, internalize it, use it as a point for meditation, then love becomes a real power. I also thank God for all the amazing people who have touched my life and pray for any people I know who are going through a difficult time emotionally or having health issues. I also send positive thoughts their way and pray for a good outcome.

Mantra 4:

I Look to a Bright Future

The three mantras you read earlier are really positive reflections on the past and present. In this final mantra, I look to and think about how bright the future can be. I find anticipating a bright future puts me in a very positive state of mind. During my run or activity, I think of all the business opportunities that lie ahead, where I am in life and where it might lead, spending time with Barb and the kids at our cottage next summer, the ability to represent Canada in the World Triathlon Championships next year. Research shows that truly happy people focus on the future and all the amazing things to look forward to. I personally find this over and over again—that happy people are really excited about the future.

You can use these mantras at different points during the day to calm your system down, de-stress, and simply to relax and calm down the monkey mind before going to bed at night. Adjust and substitute to suit your needs; they are meant as a rough guide for you to tailor to your own schedule and situation.

MENTAL SHARPNESS

We sometimes overlook the importance of staying mentally in shape as we age, as we're constantly bombarded with media messages about the rising scourge of obesity and the importance of staying physically fit. We've discussed the latter and know its importance keeping all those wheels aligned. But if you are physically fit while still being extremely stressed out, have brain fog, or are just not feeling as sharp as you once were, do not neglect the mental training you can do for yourself to reframe challenges and clear your mind. Like everything else in this book, though, take small steps. Don't go outside expecting to become one with the maple tree in your front yard and filled with love for all humankind. Just gently nudge yourself toward living a more mindful life.

The more we continue to learn as we grow older, the sharper our minds will stay.

According to Harvard Medical School, "Challenging your brain with mental exercise is believed to activate processes that help maintain individual brain cells and stimulate communication among them." By learning to play a musical instrument, learning a new skill or language, you can challenge yourself and keep mentally sharp. Even playing brain games like crossword puzzles, or those offered by the website Luminosity.com, can help keep those brain cells activated.

While the evidence as to whether brain training games strengthen the memory as we age is not yet totally conclusive, what has been found is that people who engage in new activities show improved memory performance. Experts are unsure whether people who are more mentally active begin with naturally more neural activity and continue to take part in mentally challenging activities as they age, or if the practice of engaging in these activities improves performance and memory in everyday life. Participants in one of these studies had engaged in learning digital photography and quilting, so in case you're looking for new skills to learn, these are options!

What I have found personally rewarding is investing in communication. That is, in really listening to others, meeting new people, and talking about what matters to others as well as to me. This means devoting myself to more authentic friendships, business partnerships, and relationships with others by becoming more intimate and personal. Technology can too often get in the way of our relationships as we have become overreliant on the ease of instant communication. Whether it's texting or emailing, it often seems easier than picking up the phone and having an actual conversation. We must try to not let technology control us and to make sure we are always in charge of the gadgets that try to run our lives. Your phone is a tool, not an appendage, and certainly not your boss. It should work for you—you don't work for it.

For example, make your phone 'pull' instead of 'push.' That includes changing all the settings so you don't receive any instant notifications. You have to go into each app and look for your updates or the latest emails. It eliminates the constant distraction of being alerted every 3.2 seconds when a new notification comes in. By the same token, try not to check your phone the very first thing in the morning. This puts you immediately into a reactive state. Instead, do your morning routine, as discussed earlier in the book, before engaging with technology for the first time. It will do wonders for your stress levels and make a huge difference in how you start your day.

MORE THOUGHTS ON MINDFULNESS

But what does it really mean to be mindful and increase mindfulness in your life for the benefit of your health and well-being? Mindfulness is a word that is bandied about a lot in our culture, so I want to take a minute to discuss what it really means. Mindfulness just refers to the practice of trying to be grounded in the present moment and aware of what is going on around you. If you can start by taking a few minutes, as you start or end your day—or both—to sit quietly and simply be aware, you are practicing mindfulness. No courses or self-help books required.

Productivity expert and author Tim Ferriss refers to mindfulness as the 'third leg of the stool' and probably one of the more deceivingly difficult states for Type A personalities, in particular, to occupy. But the benefits of mindfulness are too good to pass up. For one thing, being more self-aware will help you be less reactive to situations and less of a victim of the constant stress of trying to maintain a work-life balance. According to Ferriss, after just one week of mindfulness practice, "you will complain less, react less, and more effectively fill your life with what's important and valuable to you."

Leo Babauta is the founder and curator of the blog Zen Habits, one of the foremost blogs in the whole mindfulness and minimalist movement. It's a great resource. In addition to sharing his story of how he went from an overweight, in-debt smoker to a vegan long-distance runner who makes more money working for himself than he ever did before, he tackles such topics as eating, exercise, parenting, traveling, homeschooling, money management and, of course, all things mindful.

Other great resources that teach mindfulness meditation include Tara Brach, who has talks available on her website, and Sam Harris, author and speaker, who hosts the Making Sense podcast, where he also explores topics related to mindfulness and interviews our culture's thinkers, shapers, and doers. His app, Waking Up, is a step-by-step guided meditation program combined with short four-minute or five-minute lessons on the application and utility of mindfulness. Dan Harris's (good friends, no relation) *10% Happier* landed on the *New York Times* bestseller list, and for good reason. After admitting he hates the smell of patchouli, he explains how meditation changed his life and continues to make him about 10 percent happier.

In the bestselling book *Younger Next Year*, authors Chris Crowley and Henry Lodge write specifically to men 50 years old and up about how to turn their biological clocks backward and live strong and fit into their 80s and beyond. The book is a testament to the limitations we put on ourselves based on our ideas of what certain ages should look like. I can't recommend it enough. In fact, I had the privilege of hearing Chris Crowley give a talk not long ago, when we invited him to speak at my company for Advica Health clients. Chris is inspiring and drives the point home that midlife and later can, in fact, be the best time of your life if you change your mind-set and make positive choices about nutrition and fitness.

Chris also writes about the importance of finding something to be passionate about and connecting with others. Your health is important to you, and when you begin to see positive changes, so do those around you. In this way, your sphere of influence broadens. Connections with others deepen in ways not predicted. We will explore these ideas in the next chapter on community. In the meantime, let's do a little assessment. Here's your next checklist.

CHECKLIST: MINDFULNESS

Don't forget to exercise your mind, too, with these mindful practices to stay positive and focused:

- Set some mental challenges that are out of the ordinary for you, like learning a new dance, a new language, or how to play a musical instrument.
- Take time each day to be 'in the moment' and notice what's all around you.
- Start meditating five minutes every day. Every week, increase it by five minutes until you get up to 15 minutes a day.
- Devise your own positive thoughts mantra to use while exercising or starting and ending your day.
- Make a point to feel gratitude every day. Wish the best for someone else.
- Notice little things and take pleasure in them.
- Schedule down time from technology.
- Write down some goals and track your progress. (See page 174 for our Wheels of Health Daily Log you can use to track your mindfulness progress.)

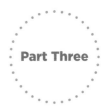

Part Three

The
Health
Action Plan

Building Communities

Your health today and the way you progress toward healthier living tomorrow affect the ultimate end goal: a long, healthy, and active life. There's no ribbon to break across a finish line, when you 'win' and are done. You never ever hit perfection. It's more like, What can I do now? How can I do that better? Is there new information I can incorporate? What else can I be doing to help myself along this health journey? To ask these questions, you have to love the commitment to living healthier. That's why it's so critical to take baby steps that slowly become habits. And also why it's often challenging to stick to changes made all at once—like an abrasive top-down management style that's forced on you, you won't love it so you're less likely to stick to it.

Taking baby steps allows you to grow into your new lifestyle in a way that develops a commitment to yourself that you're the first to notice, then your family and friends, and then the larger community. Building these communities happens organically—all of a sudden, your family is interested in that sweet potato and rice recipe you concocted in the kitchen, your friends decide to train for a 5k race, and then you're biking in Italy, talking about your blog with a reader you've never met.

Step 1:
Health Navigation

Building the community begins with you. After my wake-up call with Dr. Randy, I made a commitment to surround myself with a team of people—physicians and specialists, nutritionists and coaches who could help me navigate health strategies and opportunities and, more importantly, boost my chances of living a physical, pain-free, and full life.

Health navigation cannot be done in a silo by tapping away and chatting with Dr. Google. You need to be proactive. It involves putting names to faces and meeting with your health team.

I was grateful that I had already begun building my community years earlier when I decided to start a health navigation businesss, Advica Health. The intent was to help people navigate to the best health solutions and outcomes locally *and* globally, steering them through the endless sea of medical and instructional challenges, from getting a timely appointment to advocating for second or third opinions to working with insurance companies. Complicated medical systems require effort to find the best health solutions or secure a second opinion, and that creates a need for advocacy and support. Basically, Advica makes health care simple by advocating on our clients' behalf no matter how small or complicated the health issue—getting diagnosis, ordering prescriptions, booking specialist appointments, CT scans, ultrasounds, MRIs, etc.—and seeing real results is a measure of our success.

My work advocating on behalf of others has made me more cognizant of advocating for my own health. For example, I believe in surrounding myself with the best proactive and reactive healthcare team in order to live a very long and healthy life.

Typically, I go for an executive medical every two years. This is more than an annual physical. I get all my metrics done in a day, including multiple blood tests, ultrasounds for cancer screening and issues like hardening or weakening of the arteries, and stress tests, which determine both heart function and heart efficiency. Basically, this is an overall assessment of the whole body. I can't stress enough the importance of a thorough screening like this.

Recently, a cycling friend went for his executive medical, and discovered he had a form of ocular cancer. He was immediately scheduled for chemotherapy. If he hadn't had that executive medical, the cancer wouldn't have been found until it was untreatable. One of our clients discovered he had a shadow on his kidney during his executive medical. It turned out to be kidney cancer, but it hadn't grown to the organ's outer layer yet, which meant his prognosis was excellent. Doctors removed the kidney. That was 10 years ago, and he's been cancer-free since then.

Another client discovered a precondition during his treadmill stress test for his heart. The technicians immediately stopped the test and discovered that his heart was in terrible shape. "How long ago did you have your heart attack?" they asked him. But he had no idea he had suffered an attack, and that his heart was trying to cope with scar tissue. Once diagnosed, medication helped with the damage and his heart healed to the point where he could safely exercise again.

Prevention is often disregarded in most health-care systems and is only barely recognized in the Canadian system, so you must advocate for yourself.

This executive medical is crucial for prevention. Obviously, if you are someone with great financial resources and truly comprehensive health insurance, you have access to great health care and can afford extra tests, state of the art technology, and experimental medication, and you will be in better shape.

But what if you don't have those resources? Well, you can be self-aware and honest. Tell your doctor every little concern, every health issue you can think of, and ask questions you may have about family history and predisposition to certain medical problems. Get familiar with the types of blood panels that truly measure the status of your health. Most importantly, demand your doctor sit down with you and discuss the results thoroughly. You don't want to be given your results with an endless list of initials and terms like 'normal range,' with no context and no understanding as to what all that actually means. Have genetic tests run, and be aware of what you might be facing in the future. In health care, ignorance is not bliss.

For men, prostate cancer, lung cancer, and colon cancer are three big killers. Women need to screen for breast cancer, ovarian cancer, and lung cancer. Both sexes suffer from cardiovascular disease. Go. Get. Screened. Prevention and early detection are so critical to treatment options and outcomes. It can also work the other way. One Advica Health client had a concern show up on her annual mammogram. She was then sent for an ultrasound, which also showed there was something there, a lump. She got a third opinion from a world-renowned clinic in the U.S. Specialists there came back and told her she was fine and had nothing to worry about. No surgery to discover there was no cancer. No risk of infection. No risk from anesthesia. No more mental stress.

YOU AND YOUR HEALTH-CARE TEAM ARE PARTNERS

You are one co-partner in your health-care network; the other is your primary physician. As founder and CEO of Advica Health, I encourage our clients to select that person with care. Interview him or her, make sure that person respects your opinion, that he or she hears you, and understands you take your health seriously. You are looking for a partner in preventive health care, not a reactive medical cog in a health-care system wheel on a different track than yours. Remind your doctor that you will always seek a second opinion.

Another client was told she'd never see again in one eye, and she did, indeed, go blind in that eye. We had a second opinion from some of the best specialists in the U.S. with Harvard and Duke universities, and they came back and said there was a procedure that could be done to improve her condition. Then we found two people in Canada who were experts in doing that particular procedure, and the client had 70 percent of her eyesight restored.

Find that second opinion, always. If you are willing to go under the knife or begin a course of chemo, don't worry about hurting someone's feelings or looking unappreciative. It's your body and your life. Get another opinion.

FIND A GREAT NUTRITIONIST

Other than excellent physicians and medical specialists, find a nutritionist or dietitian you can work with who is reputable and stays current with up-to-date information. Take stock of where you are in life. If you're active, find one with a sports nutrition background. If you are a lactating mother, find one who specializes in post-partum diet and care. If you are recovering from major surgery, find one who specializes in post-surgical recovery.

I have my blood tests done two or three times a year. The blood and lipid panels, genetic test outcomes, and next steps involve a collaboration between my doctor and my nutritionist because they know me and how hard I work out. Before race season, they'll run a test, and they'll test again after a season. I meet more often with my nutritionist than I do my doctor. Why? Because given the season, the amount and kind of training I'm doing, and what I've been eating, the blood panels always reveal how I could be fueling my body differently.

> **My nutritionist will change my supplements based on my blood test results. So, if I'm training really hard, and my adrenal glands are getting shot, then she will offer a list of natural, dietary changes and supplements that will help my adrenals from becoming depleted.**

She will sit down with me and go through the results of the blood tests and tell me what I need to consume more of and what to eat less of and what levels to maintain. When I broke my ankle in a skiing accident, I sent her a note asking what I could be taking to heal more quickly. Because we have such a great relationship, and she knows me, how my body works and how I react to information, as well as what I was already taking, she was able to quickly offer a short list of additional supplements to my normal regimen to help heal my bones.

I also found it helpful to do a food sensitivity test to support some ideas I already had from paying attention to my diet. You don't have to have it done all the time. I've had my sensitivity levels tested twice. The results answer a myriad of questions, including: What foods or drinks should I not consume? How are these foods taxing my system? My results indicated I should avoid dairy. I already knew dairy left me bloated, but I didn't realize I had an actual sensitivity to it. Having a sensitivity to a food or drink is not the same as an allergy, which is an abnormal immune system reaction to something that is typically harmless to most people. A sensitivity means your system is sensitive to the substance and can cause inflammation, so the substance may affect your performance if you consume it.

The tests can be very specific. In my case, I can chomp merrily away on red peppers but I avoid green peppers. Why? They make me gassy, and I burp. Now I know my belching is not just a coincidence. A good way to use the food sensitivity test is to pay attention to the foods you should avoid—perhaps keep a food journal to support the elimination of certain food.

SEE A PHYSIOTHERAPIST OR CHIROPRACTOR AND A PHYSICAL TRAINER

Consulting a physiotherapist or chiropractor who understands your body and the stresses it undergoes is also part of building a strong team. Because I am so active, I go to my chiropractor not just for injuries but for ongoing maintenance. When I'm at home, I go once a week or once every two weeks for sessions that include massage when needed. Professional athletes have a massage every day—it's just part of their training. I see the benefit of going to help the circulation of both my blood and lymphatic systems, and it's great for muscle fatigue, as well as teaching you to listen to your body and your sore muscles. And in order to get those muscles sore, you have to exercise.

I train with a coach pretty much all year. A coach can customize a program based on your goals—for me, it's what I hope to achieve that year in terms of type, distance, and number of races I want to compete in. My coach and I train together to provide a strong foundation for my fitness goals. Then I turn to a trainer in a specific sport, running, biking, or swimming, say, for the point by point details of how to up my game.

My son Matt, for example, is my strength coach and customizes workouts for me that focus on areas I need to strengthen when I'm participating in triathlon and/or cycling races. He provides a new program every six weeks—at the end of that time, we look at the results of my workouts and then we do a reassessment and discuss options. He follows up with a new program for the next six weeks.

When I'm in triathlon season, here's how all the parts work: I spend most of my time doing cardio workouts. The trainer does an assessment, working with my chiropractor, so that several months out I also begin strength training. One assessment pointed out that my glutes and hamstrings needed work (runners have notoriously poor hamstrings!) and that I should improve my upper body strength. Instead of randomly doing a workout on my own and trying to figure out what is productive, I lean on a trainer and/or coach to interpret what my body is telling me. I let them do the translation and shape it into an effective exercise regime.

If you're going to spend time exercising, don't you want to get the most out of it?

The other element of training is psychological. It pushes you. Having a trainer with a stopwatch or telling you to do one more lift motivates you to perform at a level you might have thought was impossible on your own.

Even if that's walking one mile.

After years of working with coaches, I can just train on my own and do my own thing. But I also know a coach will sit down and say, "Okay, what are your races, and when are you racing? Here's what we need to be doing this month, next month and the month after." Coaching makes me accountable. It pushes me to perform and perform as best as I can.

If this all sounds too complicated or too expensive, or you know you have no compulsion to ever compete, you don't have to find a sports-specific trainer. Find a trainer at your gym you can work with and set up a schedule. Stick to it. Commit to it. Your baby steps might look something like this: 1) join a gym where you feel comfortable working out; 2) commit to three days a week for two months; 3) at that point, sign up for a personal trainer.

BUILD A PROACTIVE, RATHER THAN REACTIVE, TEAM

The reason I built a team of doctors, specialists, nutritionists, and coaches around me is because the health-care system in North America is predominantly reactive, not proactive. It's not really ideal health care, it's more health status quo or, you could even say, sick care.

When you're sick, you're given a treatment plan but the underlying issue isn't always explored further. Limited resources in health care, long wait times, increasing costs and access to services make it difficult for health-care providers to look ahead and assess which issues you might be facing.

Treating patients solely with prescriptions is akin to merely placing Band-Aids on a wound. Take my own situation. After my executive medical exam nine years ago, when I was told I was pre-diabetic and suffered from high cholesterol, the doctor grabbed a pen and was ready to write out several prescriptions. Statin medications, I'm sure, were at the top of his list.

That's when I asked for my three months; three months to change the course of my health. With a plan targeting my diet and fitness, I achieved my immediate health goals in one month. But here's the key: It doesn't end there. It's a process. And like anything else in modern society, that process involves institutions, red tape, rules, and conflicting information.

FIND A MEDICAL CONCIERGE SERVICE

There may be times when access to health care is limited, or your own mental and physical resources to advocate for yourself are focused on other areas, such as growing your business or family commitments. That's where a service that offers health navigation and concierge could benefit you, your family and your employees.

Here are some examples how a service such as my own company, Advica Health, has made a difference:

One of our clients, the president of a company, was suffering from painful headaches to the point where he was almost passing out. Worried he had a brain tumor, he went to see his doctor, who agreed his symptoms warranted an MRI. Our client was then given an appointment six weeks out. Meanwhile, he was worried sick about the possibility of a brain tumor. Study after study has demonstrated that the anxiety of waiting for tests and test results has a measurable effect on outcomes and overall health.

Our company was able to get him an appointment for an MRI the next day.

I want to help people take health care into their own hands. We advocate and support, and clients reap the benefits.

I got to personally experience the efficiency of our navigation service shortly after starting the company. I needed an MRI for my hamstring before Christmas, and I was on a long wait-list, perhaps as long as six months. As a result of Advica's navigation team, I was called in for an appointment on the following Tuesday and had the MRI on that Thursday, on one of the more technologically superior machines.

Instead of being at the mercy of the people at the front desk or stuck in long wait times, I got results. Fast.

In fact, one of my principles is to ensure that our team delivers care quickly, and often even virtually. This past winter, my daughter had what looked like frostbite on her toes, but she hadn't been out in the cold. Her toes were black and blue. In full dad-mode, I thought of cellulitis, a potently fatal infection. Through the company's online app, Lauren went online and spoke with a nurse. The nurse could see my daughter's toes and took pictures, then sent them to a specialist who weighed in. Was it cellulitis? Lauren was given a prescription within hours. That night, Mom and Dad slept well. Probably better than she did.

Once you have a team in place that proactively looks out for your health and helps you achieve your fitness goals, and you continue turning baby steps into habits, a slow transformation begins to take place, and not all of it is physical. You might lose some weight. You might gain some muscle. You might walk differently. But, just as important, your attitude toward achieving a healthier life will change.

And this is when your sphere of influence flexes and widens.

CHECKLIST: HEALTH NAVIGATION

- Remember, it's all about baby steps.
- Put together your own unique team of health-care practitioners.
- Get regular yearly checkups, including full blood workups.
- Invest in your own preventive health-care maintenance— don't just fix things when they're 'broken.'
- If you can, work with a physical trainer and develop a plan to get into or stay in shape.
- Learn how to be your own health-care advocate. Or partner with a team like Advica Health that can help you navigate the system and look out for your best interests.

Step 2:
Reflect Back

If you have children or work with kids, you know what a huge influence you have over them. As they grow and develop what you also find is that it's reciprocal, and then one day you find yourself being influenced by *them*. This has got to be one of the finest pleasures of parenting and parenting well. You can see this in friends, too. You offer some insight, and it comes back to you in spades. Suddenly, you're watching a film you never thought you'd enjoy or reading a book you'd normally not pick up, and it's making a lot of sense because a friend you respect recommended it.

The same can be seen when you begin turning your health around—others take notice and follow suit. Conversely, as they start down their health journey, I can learn things from them so that it becomes a sort of "movement." That's what community is: it's a give and take.

There's this idea that you are the sum of the five people you are the closest to. I'm not certain if this is right (I don't cling to absolutes), but the concept is sound. I believe we all align with people over time, and we align with people with similar interests. If I look at my group of friends, we're mostly parents to adult children and business owners, and we're all committed to making fitness and health a lifestyle.

THE FIRST INFLUENCES ARE FAMILY

When I started on this journey after receiving the really bad news from my doctor about my health situation, I went home and read a book a friend recommended called *The Hormone Diet* by Natasha Turner, a naturopathic doctor in Toronto. To simplify a very good book, she advises stripping out all the junk in your diet by detoxing for two weeks and beginning every morning with a healthy shake. You stop consuming wheat, caffeine, dairy, and alcohol. Instead, you eat vegetables and fruit and good-quality protein. Over time, you reintroduce other foods in small amounts and gauge how your body reacts.

So that's what I did. And so did Barb. Her words at the time did not reflect the level of commitment she later demonstrated. "Yeah, we should do that," was all she said initially. In fact, she became really proactive and called the number set up for the book's readers. She even got nurses involved in our dietary program. Barb became the front-runner for making sure we stayed on track. We felt and saw positive results within two weeks. We dropped weight like crazy. We made a commitment to stick with it for a while. Note the use of 'we.'

We committed to the plan for three months, eliminating foods that caused inflammation and adding whole-food options. It taught us discipline. We supported each other on our parallel journeys. And that made it fun. We were discovering something together and reaping the rewards. When I had my follow-up visit with Dr. Randy to check my blood pressure, cholesterol and insulin levels, and the results were amazing, we considered that a shared victory.

I saw the benefits derived from living well, and then Barb, who had a similar philosophy in achieving her goals, decided she was going to commit us to a higher level.

BRING THE KIDS ALONG, TOO

Next, the kids got involved. But not because we pushed them. Instead it was a symbiotic relationship.

Tim, our eldest son, had already gone vegan. He was a strong athlete at 19, and played football in college. He kept challenging me to think about a plant-based diet long before it became popular. I could see what it did for him. He was fit and lean. We started sharing all kinds of information. Then Tim introduced me to a guy named Rich Roll, one of my favorite people in the world to this day and the person who wrote this book's foreword. I started listening to The Rich Roll Podcast, and then I read his book, *Finding Ultra: Rejecting Middle Age, Becoming One of the World's Fittest Men, and Discovering Myself*, about being an athlete and eating vegan. I learned how Rich changed his life by what he put in his mouth.

I asked Rich to come to our small city of Burlington, Ontario, to speak and spread the word about the benefits of a plant-based diet and what it did to transform his life. He was impressed that we were able to fill our local performing arts center (more than 400 people showed up!) to hear his message of living a healthier life. We also assembled business leaders in our community to talk and learn about what we could do in our own companies to promote a healthier and more productive workplace for our employees. So instead of trying to help people one at a time, we had companies make bold changes in their missions by focusing more holistically on the health of their employees. This ripple effect has a much bigger impact on the health of society in general.

Tim certainly wasn't suffering from moving to a plant-based diet. In fact, Tim went on to compete with me at the World Triathlon Championships in Edmonton, as well as in Chicago, and has since changed his racing focus from running to cycling. As I was cleaning up my act, I was noticing what my kids were doing as well. I started with the baby steps. Just eating red meat when I was out or having a burger on the weekends and increasing my intake of chicken and fish. Slowly, I shifted to an entirely plant-based diet. But not all at once.

My younger son, Matt, has also followed a very healthy and fit lifestyle. He spent his early years participating in competitive sports and fitness and later focused his efforts on ski racing. He made the Canadian ski cross team and competed in the Ski Cross World Cup on a number of occasions. He has since retired from ski cross and is now very committed to CrossFit, with the goal to make the World CrossFit Games. Last year, we attended a functional fitness CrossFit competition in London, England, where he was representing Canada. Although Matt is not vegan, he eats a largely plant-based diet, and the meats and vegetables he consumes are grass-fed, wild, and organic.

Our daughter, Lauren, was the first in our family to eliminate meat from her diet at the age of 7. She has since moved to a fully vegan and plant-based diet, which she credits for making her very healthy. Lauren is also a fitness enthusiast, with her main focus on running. Last year, we watched her compete in her first ultramarathon in the pouring rain.

Lauren continues to run and train and it's a part of her overall healthy lifestyle plan.

As a family, we do many physical activities together, but the best part is the information exchange.

Now that the children are grown, nearly every week, if not every day, there's an email exchange between us. It could be a New York Times science article on fats or cholesterol, a piece lifted from a blog on running and endurance, or a video on eating plant-based foods, but we are all reading and commenting and sharing with each other.

This kind of communication keeps us focused on at least one common goal: staying healthy. This unites us in ways both practical and philosophical.

The other day I sent a picture of an aging but vibrant Dan Sullivan (founder and president of The Strategic Coach) on the treadmill to all three of my kids with the message, "Check this out. Age has no limits. Seventy-five years old." Within minutes they were telling me to write about him on my blog.

As a parent, this give-and-take between me and my children,

grown or not, can be exhilarating. It is certainly healthy and brings everyone to the table with common goals and language, while providing a way to support each other. I couldn't ask for more.

HEALTHY FRIENDSHIPS

I noticed that as I became healthier, my friends started showing an interest in running, or they'd ask me for cooking tips or why I started every day with a Wilson Shake. And they no longer laughed at my answers. They were genuinely interested. I've had friends join me on runs, taking up a sport they thought they'd never enjoy. I've had others cut back on their meat consumption. When we eat out, I never judge, but I have noticed a change in what people order. I lead by example in this small arena, but it is great to know my friendship will have a lasting impact on their health.

And again, there's the give-and-take. Many times, when people read my health blog, they send me articles or podcasts they feel will be of interest to me. I'm a serial reader, constantly ordering books that friends, readers, or acquaintances suggest to me.

WIDENING THE COMMUNITY

Over the years, I've moved from talking to my employees and colleagues about health and wellness to implementing changes. I launched a wellness program at one of my companies, and it was not uncommon for employees to have smoothies sitting on their desks in the morning.

Six years ago I started my own blog (follow kevinbradyhealth. com/blog/ to learn tips and suggestions that can improve your health). I really wanted to share my health transformation with others, hoping I could help them with their own journeys. In the beginning, I had 10 readers, and now the blog gets thousands of reads a month. Every year, I get asked to speak to a number of CEO groups on the topic of health and wellness. My intention, whether the blog has one reader or thousands, has always been the same—to share my own health journey and inspire people to take charge of their own health with gradual lifestyle adjustments.

As time goes on, you see how the work you do suddenly makes a difference and then other opportunities present themselves to do more good work. You can take those opportunities and run with them.

One of the big reasons I'm writing this book is to broaden my community—those people who are interested in their own health and want to improve it. It's the reason I speak. It's the reason I blog and Instagram and keep up to date with social media. And yes, I even send emails.

Then the community gets even bigger because people I'm influencing then return the favor and begin their own journey, surrounding themselves with people who will help them on the path to better health. When family and friends notice results, they are motivated to learn more. Then the whole environment gets involved: The workplace, the towns, the marketplace.

And suddenly you notice that the community is changing for the better.

CHECKLIST: REFLECT BACK

- Think about the five people you spend most of your time with and see if they align with your goals of how you want to live your life and where you see yourself going.
- If possible, find people to bring along with you on your new health journey.

- Try practicing new habits over smaller increments of time. For example, 24 hours, one week, three months.
- Share your own examples of your baby steps toward great health with others on social media.
- Visit AdvicaHealth.com for more health information and tips.

Step 3:

Become a Health Citizen

Being a healthy citizen, while admirable, is different than being a Health Citizen. One is insular. The other is community-minded. Of course, if everyone was healthy, our communities would be strong, and financial resources routed to care for sick people could be used in other ways. And while this is all good, I'm talking about something else. Being a Health Citizen means promoting the concept of health and wellness, almost like an ambassador. This comes with that sphere of influence, and it comes naturally.

For the last five years, I have entered a multi-day cycling race in Sardinia, Italy. Two years ago, during one of the days, I was cycling up a long mountain pass on a very hot day. It was the longest stage of the week (Grand Fondo)—over 160 kilometers in distance (picture the Tour de France). This is a stage with many long mountain climbs. Chatting with other cyclists, having the back and forth with people literally coming back and forth in my field of vision, is part of the sport.

Suddenly, this big strong guy is pumping away right next to me. First he's ahead, then I'm ahead, and we go back and forth for a while. And then he kind of looks over at me and he asks, quite matter-of-factly: "Is your name like Kevin? Brady, or Brady-health, or something like that?"

Out of a thousand participants, on a continent 4,000 miles from my own, on the side of a mountain, this guy picked me out. Because my sphere of influence broadened with my health blog. Because I was doing what I love and writing about it with passion, and he read it from the other side of the world. Turns out, he's from the Netherlands. I never saw him again. But a little miracle happened on the side of that mountain.

"I have a blog. On health," I say. "Kevin Brady Health."

"Yeah, that's it," he confirms, mostly for himself. "I follow you on Instagram."

Instagram.

All I know is that I embraced a new community, learned a bit of a new language, found common ground, and remained flexible in my thinking. I tried out new things. It started with me and my family. We borrowed from this community, and now I'm in the position of being like a mirror, reflecting this information out to others.

In short, I'm asking you to do likewise: build that community of one, then two, then many, then countless. Everyone wins.

My sphere of influence has widened so much, and surprisingly, I didn't foresee that happening at all. I've become part of a movement without ever setting out to do so.

INSPIRE OTHERS TO LIVE WELL

My message of living well aligns with the messages put out by people like my friend Rich Roll (who advocates plant-based nutrition and fitness) and Dr. Michael Greger (author of *How Not to Die*), along with many others who are all reaching their own groups, finding some overlap, and creating a movement.

Five years ago, if I went into a restaurant and tried to order a vegan dish, they kind of looked at me like I was crazy. Or it would be a big production to find the one thing I could eat on the menu, and it would probably be a salad. Today, not only can you easily order vegan and organic foods, but they're often not even listed in a separate section of the menu. You can get almond milk in your coffee and have a soy latte. This movement is so cool to witness, and it involves people of all ages and backgrounds.

Part of being a Health Citizen is listening and exchanging information and inspiration with all kinds of people. You can learn from those younger than you and be inspired by those older and vice versa. Walking into the gym and seeing people in their 80s lifting weights is inspiring. Talk to them. They're living lives worth talking about. Often you'll find they are not career gym rats. Instead, they got a wake-up call. They were challenged by a family member. They want to be able to carry groceries in from the car by themselves. Many are older women caring for grandchildren and need to be able to keep up. Some of them may have even joined the gym for the first time at the young age of 65.

I want to be one of those inspiring people. I want to spend most of my 125 years as the kind of person who helps others along their own path to fitness and health. It's like being an activist of sorts. I want to be an engaged citizen.

SUPPORT HEALTHY CHOICES BY BUYING HEALTHY

Like any engaged citizen, I vote with my wallet. I buy organic foods. I choose vegan dishes off menus. I buy the books from the thought leaders in this community. I support their work. I make sure my dollars count toward making health and wellness the first choice for people who might not otherwise be thinking of it. Promoting a grassroots effort to get a farmers market into an inner-city area, for example, would be a worthwhile endeavor. Don't have money to give? Then help develop the webpage or post on your social platforms to promote it.

You can see the health movement overtaking the marketplace. The organic section of the supermarket used to be one shelf. Now it often takes up a third of the produce, canned, and dry goods sections.

Everyone knows what quinoa is. Ten years ago, no one could spell it.

The other market area that has had to widen in order to absorb all the new participants involves physical fitness outlets like health clubs or gyms, as well as competitions. Take marathons, for instance. More than 100,000 people participate in marathons every year all across the world, and that number is doubled for half marathons. Since 1980, there has been a 32-percent increase in the number of marathon events just in the U.S., with a 255-percent increase in the number of marathon finishers. This means that not only are more people running, but more are also finishing.

And age brackets are moving up. Rather than cutting off at 70 or 75, top brackets are now going up to 100. Two years ago, I witnessed an 87-year-old competing at the World Triathlon Championships in Gold Coast, Australia. I want to be that person!

Personal accomplishment, competition, health and fitness, stress relief, and personal growth remain primary motivators for participation in the marathon, half-marathon, and long-distance running and, really, any fitness routine. This is all good news.

Just before COVID-19 hit the world, gym memberships were increasing, and boutique fitness salons were cropping up all the time. The number of gym members doubled since 2000, from 30 million to 60 million in the U.S. alone. And before you shake your head about all those people who join and don't go—well, the total number of members actively participating has grown from 60 percent to 85 percent. Europe's biggest piece of the pie in the health and fitness category is health clubs, and membership numbers there eclipse those in the U.S. It will take time for gyms to reach full capacity again but in their place, a multitude of at-home and online fitness platforms have popped up.

What does this mean? It means people care about their health. Be a Health Citizen and get out there and support the free Pilates class run at the recreation center, or join the YMCA at the corner, or commit to a membership at a health club. You are joining a wider community of people who care about their health. Be visible.

BUSINESSES SHOULD SUPPORT POSITIVE HEALTH INITIATIVES

One of the things I accomplished as a Health Citizen was to create a business that would 'increase positive patient outcomes.' That's hospital-speak for saving lives.

I just sorta fell into it... and didn't.

My passion for helping others navigate health-care hurdles dovetailed neatly with my newfound appreciation for how I could change my own body. First, I was chosen to be a kind of health coordinator in my company, and in that capacity I created wellness programs for employee plans. Next, I started Advica Heath to help people navigate to the best health solutions for them. I really took a look at the health-care industry and planned my next step. In this way, my passion carried me, but I made sure I was doing it right. Last year, I was named director of corporate health for NFP

Canada, as the company identified my passion for health and fitness in the workplace.

That commitment to health has put me on the podium on many occasions, too. I speak to groups of executives across Canada about the financial benefits of having healthy employees. The interest in creating healthy workplaces continues to grow, and there is a growing demand for my ebook titled *Return on Wellness: Turning Employee Health Into A Competitive Advantage and Bottom Line Profits*. I also consulted with other companies about what they could be doing to foster good eating habits and to integrate wellness programs into their workplaces. I listened to their answers and their concerns. None of these opportunities would have come my way if I hadn't had that wake-up call, though.

Companies who invest in promoting healthy lifestyles reap the benefits of higher productivity, lower insurance costs, higher morale, and increased workplace satisfaction. A study commissioned by a major insurance company, for example, found that for every $1 spent on employee healthy benefits program, there was a threefold return on investment. Employee morale improved by more than 50 percent, absenteeism reduced by 40 percent and productivity rose by one-third. People who have a sense of control over their health and are proactive in that area are employees who will bring that value to their work.

Wellness portals, fitness trackers, and other digital tools are enhancing workplaces, and companies are seeing real benefits to their bottom lines. To recruit and retain employees with the promise of a personalized journey to health and fitness, wellness programs have to be interactive, accessible, and meaningful. In other words, just like in business, the programs have to show measurable results. The more personalized the program, the better the results, for the employee and for the business.

But it's not just about portals and steps. It is about vending machines with healthy food, a commissary offering a wide menu of delicious meals actually cooked on-site by chefs. It's about cultivating walking groups, hosting physical events, celebrating victories. It's about creating a community where health and physical activity is valued.

And what does this bring the company who invests time, personnel, and money to structure this kind of environment? Well, a lot.

When you give people the opportunity to be physically and mentally healthier, it doesn't just cut down on sick time—it makes those employees more productive.

A study conducted by Drs. Lamar Pierce, professor of organization and strategy at Olin Business School; Timothy Gubler, assistant professor of management at the University of California-Riverside; and Ian Larkin, assistant professor of strategy at the Andersen School of Management at UCLA, used data from an industrial laundry company that provides a free, voluntary wellness program to all employees.

What they found proved stunning. Researchers compared employees who participated in the wellness plan to employees at the same company who chose not to participate. For those who did participate, not only did changes in the employees' actual productivity increase but their existing health conditions also improved. These conditions included obesity, diabetes, cholesterol, heart conditions, and also a number of self-reported behaviors of a poor diet, lack of exercise, anxiety, depression, and other mental health-related data.

The results were significant. The researchers found wellness programs boosted worker productivity by 5 percent to 11 percent compared to those who didn't participate in the program. There were measurable gains seen just from participation. Not diving in full bore, just participating. When further quantified and spread out over different variables, those figures swelled to an almost unbelievable 528 percent return on investment for the company. So, for every dollar spent, it reaped $500 in returns.

How do you calculate the ripple effect? How do you amortize and quantify the benefits to family, friends, communities, local hospitals, towns, and the personal value of being able to say, "I feel better"? By the fact that disease is down, businesses supporting health and fitness are thriving, and funds are released for literacy programs instead of paying for hospitals. Even more compelling, people are not coping with the pain and stress of chronic disease.

Once you've decided to become a Health Citizen, speak up to your employer. Ask if you can volunteer to coordinate a walking group or a vegan lunch recipe-swap potluck on Wednesdays. Challenge Human Resources to expand its health and wellness program. If you are in a leadership position, start making small changes that will support wellness at your company. Models for wellness programs are changing and changing fast. There is so much you can do for your employees and for the bottom line. Just remember to let the employees buy into the concept. That's the key to participation.

PRACTICE PREVENTION

When I started Advica Health, the company was focused primarily on reactionary health. For example, if someone had a heart attack, we had to figure out how can we get him or her to the right hospital and the best care within parameters like insurance or limited services available.

We focused on making sure clients received the best treatments or health care, and by coordinating a team to help them navigate the system, created a health-care concierge service. And that's originally how the program was started: to essentially get clients the best health solutions locally and around the world, depending on what their health circumstances were.

As our company grew, it became alarmingly clear that we needed to be more than reactive. Because I've witnessed the personal benefits of preventive health, we expanded our mission and now we "serve the health needs of individuals, families, and communities through a holistic philosophy rooted in our fundamental understanding of human beings." That holistic philosophy is about prevention and improvement, not merely attending to a client when there's a crisis.

In order to realize that mission, we facilitate appointments with clients for nutritionists, dietitians, genetic testing, food sensitivity testing, and baseline testing for diabetes and blood pressure. If the expectation is you're never getting off those high blood pressure meds your doctor prescribed, then you won't. Apparently, you're always going to have high blood pressure.

But if you change your diet and begin exercising, you could potentially be off your medication in as little as a month.

The average Westerner takes more than 10 prescription pills over a limited duration by the age of seventy. A third of the elderly take more than five prescription drugs daily. Anything past number five and you're in the polypharmacy realm. In that world, you have a one in three chance of taking two or more drugs that will negatively interact with each other. Doing the math is scary.

On top of that, we have ready access to over-the-counter meds that may also react with prescription drugs. Sometimes, a medication may conteract with another drug and, therefore, reduce the effects of that medication or cause other issues. It's like once a prescription is written for a 'chronic' condition, it's a done deal. No going back.

PREVENTING CHRONIC CONDITIONS IS THE BEST APPROACH TO LONG-TERM HEALTH

Relying on drugs alone will never be as effective as a strategy that also integrates a non-pharmaceutical component that includes a whole-food diet and exercise routine. Why not promote that?

Advica Health helps companies by setting up programs that will help employees prevent chronic conditions instead of just reacting to them. We're trying to avoid the polypharmacy problem decades in advance. Every quarter there's a new challenge.

For example, recently employees under our plan did a Mount Everest virtual 'hike' for 5,000 steps or 30 minutes of exercise. They used wearables or Apple Watches or Fitbits that all fed into the same program, where participants also monitored their food intake. This program becomes a one-stop shop, where each employee's data is in one place. We've witnessed real results. Challenge after challenge, the companies that put these programs in place saw improvements not only in employee productivity, but also in achieving their overall health goals within 60 days.

I speak regularly to groups of CEOs about driving profits through corporate wellness initiatives, and instituting best practices for launching this kind of wellness program for their companies. I'm initially met with some skepticism, but it quickly turns to interest once they see the evidence I'm able to present.

It's hard to argue with facts.

Enlarging your sphere of influence, leading by example, is a gift you can give to others. Your health begins with you. It doesn't have to end with you, however. Building a legacy is a long-term commitment. Let yours be a positive force for others, and you leave the planet—decades from now—a better place.

CHECKLIST: BECOME A HEALTH CITIZEN

- Identify your influences and use them to motivate your baby steps.
- Pinpoint your spheres of influence, where *you* could make a difference.
- Listen to others and their health concerns.
- If you're in a position to authorize programs, begin to make changes in your company or family.
- If you're an employee, talk to human resources, as well as your boss, and bring resources with you to back up ideas you may have for improving the quality of health in the workplace. One-hour lunch walk, anyone? Vegan day?
- Share what you know with others in conversation, on blogs, in groups.
- Be a Health Citizen.

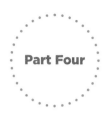

Part Four

Resources, Routines & Recipes

Build Your Resources

Now that you have come this far in the book, I hope you really understand how perfection is the enemy of progress. It's also the enemy of productivity. I want you to put down this book with a solid feeling of "I've got this." You're going to apply the 80/20 Rule in your life and take baby steps every day toward your health and wellness goals. Don't get hung up on the details of whether to add kale *or* avocado to your morning shake, or whether to walk three miles on the treadmill *or* two miles on the hiking trail. Honestly, those kinds of details are not important. What is important is the commitment to making healthy choices every day.

My other parting advice for you is to go for the low-hanging fruit when you're starting out. Meaning, it may be easier for you to cut out eating pizza for lunch every day rather than waking up half an hour earlier to make a healthy shake. Maybe it's easier to take the stairs at work instead of the elevator. I think you get the idea. Find those effortless opportunities, and you're then more than 25 percent on the way to your 80 percent.

The point is, we're all works in progress. I have not mastered this by any means—I'm continually tweaking, hacking, learning, and growing. I also continue to challenge myself because I enjoy the process.

I enjoy feeling more fit than I was 20 years ago. Do I mess up sometimes? Of course I do. But I hit the reset button and start again. Try not to beat yourself up and think that all is lost if you revert to old, less-than-optimal habits. You start by trying to change one thing—today you do one push-up, tomorrow maybe it's two. Today you replace your mid-afternoon snack of Doritos with a handful of almonds and dried fruit. I guarantee you'll feel better and more sated. Use the "Follow Routines" section that follows to give you some ideas of sample recipes and what my morning and nighttime routines look like.

Ultimately, there are no rules about what your life has to look like or that say your health should necessarily decline as you grow older. In fact, the opposite can be true. But it is first up to you to realize you do have the power to transform your health and your life.

Now that we've come full circle, you have all of the basic components of your Wheels of Health, which will help propel you toward a healthier, more vibrant you. You've learned that eating right, exercising regularly, sleeping well, and learning to be more mindful are the spokes of your wheel. When these are all aligned properly, it will be easy to keep rolling forward toward building a better life, community, and sense of well-being. Now that you're aware of healthier food choices, you have free will to choose more wisely. But when one spoke gets out of whack, it may make your wheel wobbly. As I said at the beginning of the book, keeping these four segments roughly aligned at 4 or 5 is your roadmap to peak condition or, more simply, better health. But again, don't forget our 80/20 Rule while exploring each spoke of your wheel. It all starts with those baby steps!

Follow Routines

I know I'm the kind of person who thrives on routine. I try to schedule my days the same way each week. For example, on Mondays, you'll find me in the office having meetings. Tuesdays through Thursdays I'm out of the office, meeting with clients. Then on Fridays, I work *on* the business rather than *in* the business. What this means is that I tend to work on high-level strategic projects instead of on a client's plan. The goal of my businesses is to help people lead more healthy, energized, and productive lives.

As I've mentioned throughout this book, I've found the most important strategy for improving health is to take baby steps. People try to take on way too much at once, and as a result, they fail—or more to the point, they feel like they failed, and so give up too soon. People often make unrealistic commitments they ultimately can't live up to. Someone who wants to lose 25 pounds goes on a restricted diet and embarks on a seven-day-a-week gym schedule. Neither is sustainable.

So incorporate one small change at a time. Once you've turned that change into a habit, shift your focus, and commit to another change. By incorporating this strategy, all of those baby steps accumulate over time, while overall health dramatically improves. I meet with my nutritionist/dietitian every quarter. This allows me to make one small change, a small commitment for the next quarter, and improve one aspect of my health.

HERE ARE SOME EXAMPLES OF BABY STEPS YOU MIGHT COMMIT TO TAKING IN YOUR OWN LIFE:

- I am going to go to the gym three times a week.
- I am going to go to bed and get up at the same time every day, therefore ensuring I'm getting a consistent amount of sleep.
- I am going to have meat only once a week.
- I am going to have a Wilson Shake every weekday morning.
- I am going to have five servings of fruits or vegetables every day.
- I am going to walk 5,000 to 10,000 steps a day.
- I am going to try meditation techniques and see what works for me.
- I am going to go for a comprehensive medical exam once a year.

If you work on improving one thing at a time it's much easier, as you're only changing and focusing on a single habit.

Besides thriving on routines, I love tracking results. In business and in my personal life, I can keep to my own 80/20 Rule (see page 26 for more information) because I update my Wheels of Health Daily Log (see page 172) every night. I track what exercise I did for the day, along with what I ate, how many hours I slept, and the quality of my sleep. Then, I have a box where I note my assessment of how I did: satisfactory, fairly well, or excellent. I make a note of what I can do to improve for the next day. There's an old saying, "What you measure is what you succeed at." I live this. I do this every night, and at the end of the week, I add up my hours of working out and sleeping and see how I can improve going forward.

These are some of the strategies and routines that help me feel in control, centered, and mindful. What I do may not work for you, but that's the point. I've found what works for me, and hopefully, you will experiment, be inspired by some of these ideas, and find your own way. There are hundreds of apps and books out there. If you need help figuring out a way to clear your mind, find one that speaks to you (I also recommend my top picks on page 175).

Morning Routine Checklist:

- Get daylight on your eyeballs as soon as you wake up
- Filtered warm lemon water
- Morning workout or easy exercise
- The Wilson (morning) Shake
- Vitamins
- A cold shower
- Organic Americano coffee
- Intermittent fasting at least once a week

Nighttime Routine Checklist:

- No screens or TV within an hour of bed
- Put on screen filtering to block blue rays
- No TV while in bed
- Limit alcohol
- Nightly supplement routine
- Teaspoon of honey
- Make your room as dark as possible
- Gratitude—give thanks for three things that happened during the day

PLAN TO EAT WELL

Fear has no place in a kitchen! The kitchen is truly the heart of the home, a place to linger and talk about the day, a place to laugh, a place to plan, and above all, a place to create meals. Ours is organized with routines that accommodate hectic work and school schedules. The blender is always on the counter with fun brushes to clean it, so no one's stuck with dried-on smoothie to pry off. Food is prepared in advance and stored. Snacks are fixed to grab and go. The kitchen, prep areas, and food storage all need to be functional.

I have everything laid out, so it's easy and quick for me to access foods and prep meals. For example, I have all the ingredients portioned out beforehand for my morning shake in the freezer, the fridge, and in my cupboard with all my supplements. Therefore, it literally takes me about one minute to put all the ingredients together for my morning shake.

Planning is critical. At least for me. When we go shopping, Barb and I ensure that we get the very best ingredients for simple meal preparation, including staples like rice, organic fruits and vegetables, quinoa, lentils, almond butter, nuts and seeds, and organic and gluten-free crackers.

On days when I'm traveling to meet with clients, I set out containers and fill them with simple ingredients. For example, I'll take some cooked rice and sweet potato from the fridge (already prepared), add some arugula or spinach to it, add some nutritional yeast and hot sauce, and put it in a container to eat on the road or to take to work with me. This is a two-minute job. The result is that I'm able to have a very healthy plant-based lunch wherever I am. To plan for this means that I have to make sure I cook enough for several lunches the night before.

Routines are important, as well. Here's a bird's-eye view of a typical Sunday night.

Every Sunday night, we prep our food for the week (see how I like to plan?). This includes baking many types of vegetables, such as squash, zucchini, yams, cauliflower and potatoes, and a pot full of whole-grain rice (thanks to Barb!). From these staples, Barb makes squash soup, adds the veggies to salads, or makes a rice bowl, burritos or wraps. This is a great way to skip the dishes every night and create your own magic in the kitchen with what's available. During the week, only assembly is required.

SWING WITH THE SEASONS

It's good to stay in touch with the seasons when it comes to food and food prep. Menus can mirror what's going on in your garden or how carefully you preserved foods from other seasons. The seasons are a natural routine in themselves and create a rhythm reflected on our plates.

I instinctively prefer different foods at different times of the year.

Spring is good for returning to those great farmers markets. Baby greens are everywhere, ushering in both spring and summer, and we eat lots of fresh garden vegetables. I find that with all the fresh ingredients available I eat salads almost every day in the spring and summer. As late summer approaches, we turn to fresh tomatoes and incorporate more of those into our meals. In the fall and winter, I tend to eat and crave more cooked vegetables, vegan pasta, and vegetable-based warm soups. I think the key message here is that you should try to eat according to the current season and, if possible, eat food that is sourced locally. For example, when I buy apples, I always try to buy local Canadian apples or at least from as close to home as possible. Therefore, if the closest fresh organic produce is from the U.S., then I will choose that over something from overseas.

In terms of experimenting, if everything is premade, chopped, cooked, and ready to go, then it's very easy to mix things up. For example, last night we had a great stir-fry. Barb took all the vegetables in our produce drawer and cooked them in a wok with premade long-grain brown rice, and in a matter of minutes we had a very healthy and filling stir-fry full of goodness. Today I'm taking the leftovers to work and will have it for lunch. It doesn't get much easier than this!

Summer brings an explosion of fresh vegetables and fruits. We tend to buy as much as we can that's fresh and organic and freeze it for later use. For example, often we will overbuy fresh strawberries or blueberries and then freeze a bunch of them to throw in our shakes in the morning. In the winter months, I buy frozen organic fruits and vegetables to use in my shakes, and they are very fresh and full of nutrients. Often they were frozen right after they were picked, so we're actually eating fresh produce. The end of summer is a great time to stop by farms for bushels of apples and tomatoes. Clean them, dry them, roast them in the oven and then blend them up and freeze by the quart for sauces.

Fall is squash time. Did you know you don't have to cut your squash or yams before baking? Just wash and poke once or twice with a fork to let the heat out while cooking. I usually cut the end of the yams off and sprinkle with pink Himalayan salt and oregano and rosemary and roast them. And then roast a lot of them for later. Fall is the time for prep and storage.

When September hits, I don't throw out my herbs, but rather dry them for winter use. This is what you see in Canada. You can buy herbs still on the stalks in grocery stores during the winter, too. Barb makes homemade jams, pickles, and beets. For example, we went strawberry picking while at the cottage and, from that harvest, Barb made a batch of healthy strawberry jam that we can consume all year long.

And in the dead of winter, there are those frozen blueberries you picked in the summer to enjoy, rich soups you can cook ahead, and all of a sudden the slow cooker becomes your best friend.

Recipes

I believe that healthy, nutritious, plant-based eating not only makes you feel fantastic, but can taste delicious, too. The kitchen is where my family and I spend most of our time together, experimenting with new recipes and indulging in old favorites. Leading a healthy life means balanced and enjoyable meals so that you'll ultimately feel energized and ready to take on a new day.

If you do nothing else for your health, start the day with my first recipe, The Wilson Shake. It's an all-time favorite, happily named after my dog Wilson, who lived to the ripe old age of 18! Every morning, without fail, Wilson would accompany me to the kitchen and beg for a taste.

In this section, you'll find a selection of recipes that are often served at my table, some of which have been curated from my favorite recipe developers and food bloggers. You'll find a delicious assortment of plant-based dishes, including a power breakfast, vegan main dishes, warming soups, fresh salads, versatile sides, dressings and dessert ideas for you, your family and friends to savor. I hope you enjoy!

Power Breakfast .... page 126
Vegan Mains .... page 128
Soups, Salads & Sides .... page 152
Desserts .... page 168

THE WILSON SHAKE

Serves 2-4

- 1 cup frozen organic fruits (strawberries, raspberries, blueberries, mixed berries—see TIPS)
- 1-2 cups frozen or fresh organic vegetables (see TIPS)
- 1 to 2 tbsp spirulina
- 1 tsp chlorella
- 1 tsp maca powder
- 1 scoop plant-based protein powder
- 1 or 2 tbsp chia, flax or hemp seeds
- 1 tsp ground cinnamon
- 1 tsp turmeric
- ½ tsp vitamin C powder

When training or working out a lot, I add:

- 1 tsp glutamine
- 1 tsp creatine

Add all ingredients to a blender. Fill blender with enough filtered water to cover the top of the ingredients and blend away until smooth. Enjoy!

TIPS

- If I have organic fresh fruits, I often throw some in as well.
- I mix up the vegetables, depending on what's in the fridge, such as spring mix lettuce, spinach or arugula.

The following ingredients address the following nutritional needs:

- Spirulina for antioxidants
- Chlorella for antioxidants
- Maca powder for energy and recovery
- Seeds for healthy fats and fiber
- Cinnamon for blood pressure and cholesterol
- Turmeric to reduce inflammation
- Vitamin C powder to boost the immune system
- Glutamine to assist in recovery and reduce inflammation
- Creatine to assist in recovery

VEGAN MAC & CHEESE
Serves 4

¾ cup raw cashews

1 pkg (10 oz/280 g) brown rice or quinoa pasta shells
  (spirals or elbows)

2 cups butternut squash soup

1 cup vegetable broth

3 heaping tbsp nutritional yeast

1 tbsp vegan Dijon mustard

2 tsp garlic powder

½ tsp turmeric

½ tsp salt

Topping:

1 cup whole wheat or gluten-free bread crumbs

2 tbsp nutritional yeast

2 tbsp olive or avocado oil

½ tsp salt

1. Soak cashews in hot water for 20 minutes, until softened. Drain cashews.

2. In a pot of boiling water, cook pasta according to package directions just until al dente (still firm to the bite). Drain and rinse with cold water; set aside.

3. Preheat oven to 400°F. Lightly grease a 7 x 11-inch baking dish. Place reserved cashews, squash soup, vegetable broth, nutritional yeast, mustard, garlic powder, turmeric and salt in a high-powered blender. Set aside.

4. For the topping, stir together all ingredients until well combined; set aside.

5. In a large bowl, mix together drained pasta and cashew sauce and pour into prepared pan. Sprinkle topping evenly over top and cover with foil.

6. Bake for 20 minutes. Remove foil and bake for another 15 minutes or until golden on top. Let stand for 5 minutes before serving.

Excerpted from Protein Ninja by Terry Hope Romero

QUINOA RISOTTO

Serves 2-4

1½ cups quinoa

3 cups vegetable broth, divided

1 clove garlic, minced

½ onion, chopped

1 cup chopped broccoli florets

1 cup sliced mushrooms

1 tsp chopped fresh parsley

Salt and freshly ground black pepper to taste

1. Rinse quinoa in a fine mesh colander under running water. Drain.

2. Combine quinoa with 2⅔ cups vegetable broth in saucepan. Bring mixture to a boil over medium-high heat; decrease heat to a gentle simmer. Cook until quinoa has absorbed all the liquid, about 12 to 18 minutes.

3. In a skillet, put remaining ⅓ cup vegetable broth, bring to a boil and add garlic and onion, cooked until the onion is translucent. Add broccoli and mushrooms and sauté until they are tender-crisp. Stir in cooked quinoa, parsley, and salt and pepper to taste.

4. Mix well and serve hot.

Excerpted from Quinoa 365 by Patricia Green

RATATOUILLE

Serves 2-4

1 tbsp avocado oil

1 onion, chopped

1 large eggplant, diced

2 cloves garlic, finely chopped

2 medium zucchini

1 red bell pepper, chopped

1 can (14 oz/398 ml) diced tomatoes

Salt and freshly ground black pepper

¾ cup quinoa

1 cup hot water

1 bunch chopped fresh parsley

1. In a large saucepan, heat avocado oil over medium-high heat and cook onion until softened and translucent.

2. Add eggplant and cook for 5 to 10 minutes. Add garlic, zucchini, red pepper and canned tomatoes; season with salt and freshly ground black pepper. Cover and simmer for 15 minutes or until vegetables are tender.

3. Stir quinoa with the hot water and pour into saucepan. Toss gently and simmer for 15 minutes or until quinoa is cooked. Season to taste. Sprinkle with parsley just before serving.

Excerpted from Cooking With Quinoa By Rena Patten

VEGAN BURGER PATTIES

Makes 23-24 vegan patties

¾ cup ground flax seeds

⅓ cup warm water

2 cups toasted sunflower seeds

4 cups rolled oats, processed into a flour

4 tsp chili powder

4 tsp dried oregano

4 tsp ground cumin

4 tsp fine sea salt

Freshly ground black pepper

4 cups grated carrots

2 cups chopped onions

2 cloves garlic, chopped

4 cans (19 oz/540 ml each) black beans, drained and rinsed

Avocado oil

1. Combine ground flax seed and warm water and set aside for 10 minutes or until thickened.

2. In a large mixing bowl, combine toasted sunflower seeds, oat flour, chili powder, dried oregano, ground cumin, sea salt and black pepper. Mix together and set aside.

3. Using a food processor, pulse together carrots, onions and garlic. Process or mash black beans into a paste, leaving a few beans intact; combine with vegetables and flax seed mixture. Adjust seasonings to taste. Mix well until combined.

4. Using ½ cup measuring at a time, shape mixture into patties with slightly greased hands (using avocado oil). Place the patties on a parchment-lined baking sheets and freeze for at least an hour before grilling. Store remaining burgers in between parchment paper in resealable freezer bags.

5. When ready to cook, preheat grill to medium heat. Place burgers directly on grill and cook for about 10 minutes, flipping in between until lightly browned.

TIP

- These burgers freeze well; cook directly on a grill from frozen.

Adapted from The Oh She Glows Cookbook by Angela Liddon

VEGETABLE LASAGNA

Serves 4-6

Filling:

2½ cups cauliflower florets, cut into small pieces

1½ cups raw cashews, chopped

1 tbsp chopped fresh basil

2 tsp salt

Freshly ground black pepper

1 large eggplant, cut into small cubes

1 lb cremini mushrooms, trimmed and thinly sliced

1 clove garlic, minced

1 lb zucchini, cut into small cubes

Olive oil

Salt

12 no-boil brown rice lasagna noodles

Tomato Sauce:

1 can (28 oz/796 ml) crushed tomatoes

1 can (28 oz/796 ml) diced tomatoes

¼ cup chopped fresh basil

2 cloves garlic

¼ tsp red pepper chili flakes

½ tsp salt

1. For the filling: Combine 12 cups water, cauliflower, cashews and salt into a large saucepan. Bring to a boil and cook until cauliflower is fork-tender, about 20 minutes. Save ¼ cup broth for later use before draining. Let cool slightly.

2. In a food processor, combine cauliflower mixture, ¼ cup cauliflower broth, basil, salt and freshly ground black pepper. Process until smooth. Set aside.

3. Preheat oven to 450°F. Toss eggplant, mushrooms and garlic in a large bowl and sprinkle with a little bit of olive oil and salt, then spread on a parchment-lined baking sheet. Roast eggplant and mushrooms for about 15 minutes. Add zucchini into eggplant-mushroom mixture and roast for another 15 to 20 minutes, until zucchini and eggplant are tender and mushrooms are lightly browned. Set aside.

4. For the tomato sauce: Combine crushed tomatoes, diced tomatoes, basil, garlic, red pepper flakes and salt into a blender. Blend until smooth and set aside.

5. In a 13 x 9-inch baking pan, spread some tomato sauce over bottom of dish. Arrange 4 noodles on top. Spread some cauliflower filling over noodles followed by half of roasted vegetables and spread ¾ cup tomato sauce. Repeat layering with 4 noodles, cauliflower filling, remaining vegetables and ¾ cup tomato sauce. Arrange remaining 4 noodles on top spread some cauliflower filling and cover completely with remaining tomato sauce.

6. Preheat oven at 375°F. Cover dish with aluminum foil and bake for 45 to 50 minutes.

7. Let cool a little before serving.

Excerpted from Vegan for Everybody by America's Test Kitchen

VEGETARIAN SHEPHERD'S PIE

Serves 4-6

1 tsp avocado oil

½ onion, diced

2 cloves garlic, minced

2 carrots, diced

2 celery stalks, diced

1 cup sliced button mushrooms

¾ tsp sea salt

1 tsp dried thyme

½ tsp paprika

Pinch cayenne pepper

Freshly cracked black pepper

1 can (5.5 oz/156 ml) tomato paste

2 cups vegetable broth + more

1 cup canned black beans, drained and rinsed

1 cup frozen peas

4 cups mashed potatoes

1. In a large skillet over medium heat, heat avocado oil and cook onion and garlic until until onion is softened and translucent.

2. Add carrots and celery to the skillet and continue to cook until celery begins to soften slightly, about 5 minutes.

3. Stir in mushrooms, salt, thyme, paprika, cayenne and black pepper. Continue cooking until mushrooms have fully softened. Add tomato paste. Stir mixture until vegetables are fully coated with tomato paste.

4. Add vegetable broth, stirring to dissolve the paste from the bottom of the skillet. Allow broth to come up to a simmer, at which point it will become slightly thicker.

5. Stir in black beans and frozen peas; allow mixture to heat through. You can add more broth if the sauce is too thick for you.

6. Preheat oven to 400°F. Pour vegetable mixture into a casserole dish. Spread the mashed potatoes overtop vegetables.

7. Bake in preheated oven for 15 minutes, or until everything is heated through.

8. To brown top, turn on oven broiler and watch closely until the top has browned to your liking.

VEGAN WRAP

Serves 2-4

1 cup sliced red bell peppers

1 cup sliced onion

1 cup sliced celery

1 cup sliced mushrooms

2 tbsp coconut oil, divided

Salt and freshly ground black pepper

1 head cauliflower, chopped

1 cup panko crumbs

4 large whole-grain tortilla wraps

Dijon mustard

Vegan mayonnaise

Dairy-free cheese

Hot Sauce (such as Frank's Red Hot)

Cilantro

1. Preheat oven to 375°F.

2. In a large bowl, combine red peppers, onion, celery and mushrooms. Toss with half the oil and season with salt and freshly ground black pepper to taste. Place vegetables in a single layer on a parchment-lined baking sheet and bake for 20 to 25 minutes.

3. In another large bowl, toss cauliflower with remaining oil. Add greased cauliflower into a resealable bag with panko crumbs; seal bag and shake to evenly coat. Place coated cauliflower on a parchment-lined baking sheet and bake in preheated oven for 30 minutes.

4. When vegetables are almost done cooking, warm up wraps on a non-stick baking sheet in a warm oven for a few minutes.

5. Fill each tortilla wrap with desired vegetables and condiments down the center: Spread with Dijon, mayonnaise, vegetables, cheese, hot sauce and cilantro. Tuck in vegetables while rolling and enjoy.

TIP

- You can add 1 tbsp curry powder to cauliflower, if desired.

QUICK STIR-FRY, TACOS OR WRAPS

Serves 2-4

2 tbsp avocado oil

2 carrots, sliced

2 celery stalks, sliced

1 head broccoli, sliced into ½-inch steaks

3 zucchini, sliced in rounds and cut in half

1 onion, sliced

2 red bell peppers, sliced

Salt and freshly ground black pepper

1 tsp curry powder or cumin (optional)

1 cup canned black beans, rinsed and drained

6 taco shells or 6 large tortilla wraps

Garnishes:

1 cup radishes, sliced

1 cup chopped jalapeño peppers

1 cup chopped fresh cilantro

Store-bought salsa

1 cup dairy-free cheese

1. In an extra-large skillet, heat oil on medium-high heat. Add carrots, celery and broccoli. Stir-fry until vegetables are starting to soften, about 5 minutes. Toss in zucchini, onion and red peppers; cook 5 more minutes until all vegetables are tender. Season with salt and freshly ground black pepper and curry, if using.

2. Stir in black beans and toss well.

3. Serve vegetable-bean mix with tacos or tortilla wraps. Fill/roll with mixture and top with garnishes of your choice, including radishes, jalapeños, cilantro, salsa and cheese.

TIPS:

- If there are any leftovers, add rice noodles the next night for a delicious stir-fry—it always tastes better the next day!

- Get ahead of meal prepping by cutting your veggies the night before.

VEGAN PIZZA
Serves 2-4

Store-bought organic tomato sauce or pizza sauce

Store-bought or prepared pizza crust

1 tbsp extra-virgin olive oil

¼ cup each: chopped onions, zucchini, red bell peppers and
mushrooms

1 cup shredded dairy-free cheese

¼ cup halved cherry tomatoes

Optional: nutritional yeast and red pepper chili flakes

1. Preheat oven to 450°F.

2. Spread tomato sauce as needed on crust.

3. In a medium skillet, heat oil on medium-high heat. Add onions,
zucchini, red peppers and mushrooms. Toss and cook for 3 to 4 minutes
or just until softened.

4. Scatter vegetables evenly over sauce and top with cheese and cherry
tomatoes.

5. Bake in preheated oven on middle oven rack for 10 to 12 minutes or
until crust is golden.

6. Sprinkle with nutritional yeast and red pepper chili flakes, if using,
before serving.

TIP

- When we can't make our own pizza crust, we usually pick
  up a premade crust from the freezer of our grocer's health-
  food section. A cauliflower pizza crust also works well
  here. Alternatively, you could also use whole wheat wraps.

JAPANESE STIR-FRY
Serves 2-4

1 tbsp coconut oil
1 cup chopped onions
1 cup thinly sliced carrots
1 cup sliced celery
1 cup sliced mushrooms
3 or 4 ears corn on the cob, steamed
1 cup snow peas
3 mini bok choy, separated and roughly chopped
1 cup cherry tomatoes
16 oz (454 g) rice noodles
3 to 4 tbsp sesame sauce, oyster sauce or soy sauce

1. In a large skillet, heat oil on high heat. Add onions, carrots, celery and mushroom. Stir mixture continuously for about 5 minutes or until vegetables are tender-crisp (don't overcook them).

2. Cut corn off cob in long strips. Add to skillet and toss well.

3. Add snow peas and bok choy. Toss and cook mixture, with lid, for 5 more minutes. Add tomatoes and remove from heat (you want the tomatoes just to warm so they don't break apart).

4. In the meantime, prepare the rice noodles: Soak noodles in hot water for about 5 to 10 minutes until noodles have softened.

5. Add sesame sauce to vegetable mix. Toss and serve hot over drained noodles.

PANKO CAULIFLOWER WINGS

Serves 2-4

2 large heads cauliflower

3 tbsp coconut oil

2 cups panko crumbs

Salt and freshly ground black pepper

Buffalo hot sauce or barbeque sauce for serving

1. Cut cauliflower to the size of chicken wings. Preheat oven to 375°F.

2. In a large bowl, add cauliflower wings; sprinkle with coconut oil and toss until pieces are well coated.

3. Add greased cauliflower into a resealable bag with panko crumbs; seal bag and shake to coat evenly.

4. Place coated cauliflower on a parchment-lined baking sheet and bake for 30 minutes. Sprinkle with salt and freshly ground black pepper.

5. Bake for 45 minutes or until lightly golden.

6. Serve drizzled with buffalo hot sauce or barbeque sauce.

TIP

- These cauliflower wings work great in wraps, too.

VEGETABLE STIR-FRY WITH CASHEWS

Serves 2-4

2 tbsp coconut oil

1 cup sliced onions

1 cup sliced yellow bell peppers

3 medium carrots, thinly sliced in strips

3 celery stalks, thinly sliced

3 medium zucchini, halved and sliced

1 cup sliced mushrooms

16 oz (450 g) rice noodles

1 can (19 oz/540 ml) red kidney beans, rinsed and drained

1 can (19 oz/540 ml) chickpeas, rinsed and drained

Salt and freshly ground black pepper

¼ cup chopped fresh cilantro

¼ cup raw or toasted cashews

1. In a large wok or skillet, heat oil on medium-high heat. Add onions, yellow peppers, carrots celery, zucchini and mushrooms. Stir mixture continuously for about 5 minutes or until vegetables are tender-crisp (don't overcook them).

2. In the meantime, cook rice noodles according to package directions.

3. Add red kidney beans and chickpeas to vegetable mixture; toss until fully combined.

4. Drain rice noodles and add to wok.

5. Serve with cilantro and cashews—either right from the pan or on a serving platter.

VEGAN CHILI
Serves 4-6

1 tbsp coconut oil

1 cup chopped onions

1 cup chopped red or green bell peppers

1 cup chopped mushrooms

1 cup chopped celery

3-4 zucchini, sliced and cut into half-moons

2 cans (28 oz/796 ml each) whole peeled tomatoes, coarsely chopped (with liquid)

1 can (28 oz/796 ml) diced tomatoes

1 can (5.5 oz/156 ml) tomato paste

1 can (19 oz/540 ml) chickpeas, drained and rinsed

1 can (19 oz/540 ml) red kidney beans, drained and rinsed

1 can (19 oz/540 ml) black beans, drained and rinsed

1 can (14 oz/398 ml) baked brown beans in tomato sauce

3 tbsp Worcestershire sauce or coconut aminos

4 tbsp chili powder

2 handfuls fresh spinach

Optional: Hot sauce (such as Sriracha), dairy-free cheese or nutritional yeast

1. In a large pot, heat oil on medium-high heat. Add onion and cook until softened, about 2 minutes. Add peppers, mushrooms, celery and zucchini; cook for 3 to 4 minutes.

2. Add tomatoes with liquid and tomato paste; stir until paste is dissolved. Bring mixture to a boil.

3. Add chickpeas, red kidney beans, black beans and baked beans. Stir until combined. Season with Worcestershire sauce and chili powder. Reduce heat to a simmer and cook for 3 hours on slow simmer.

4. Add spinach and cook just until it wilts.

5. Stir in hot sauce, cheese or nutritional yeast, if using, just before serving. Serve with toasted whole-grain bread, pita or wrap.

LOADED SWEET POTATO

Serves 6

4 medium sweet potatoes

1 tbsp avocado oil

1 onion

1 clove garlic, minced

¼ tsp chili powder + more for garnish

¼ tsp ground cumin + more for garnish

1 can (19 oz/540 ml) black beans, drained and rinsed

Salt and freshly ground black pepper

Freshly squeezed lime juice

2 green onions, thinly sliced

Avocado Cilantro Cream:

½ cup fresh cilantro, stems removed

1 clove garlic

1 medium ripe avocado

4 tsp freshly squeezed lime juice

1 tbsp water

Salt to taste

Vegan Sour Cream (optional, see page 167)

1. Preheat oven to 400°F. Line a baking sheet with parchment paper. Poke several holes into each potato. Place on a baking sheet and roast for 60 to 75 minutes, depending on size, until flesh is tender and easily pierced with a fort in the center. Let cool for 5 to 10 minutes.

2. Make the avocado cilantro cream. In a food processor, process cilantro and garlic until minced. Add remaining ingredients and process until smooth.

3. In a medium skillet, heat oil over medium heat and cook onion and garlic until onion is softened. Stir in chili powder, cumin and black beans; cook for 2 minutes. Add salt, pepper and lime juice and stir again to combine.

4. Assemble the sweet potatoes. Slice each potato in half lengthwise. With a knife, score the flesh in a crisscross pattern. Gently mash flesh with a fork to fluff. Season with salt and freshly ground black pepper to taste. Dollop a tablespoon of Avocado Cilantro Cream and black bean mixture. Garnish with green onions, a pinch of chili powder and cumin. Serve with Vegan Sour Cream, if using.

Adapted from The Oh She Glows Cookbook by Angela Liddon

SIMPLE VEGGIE PASTA WITH OLIVE OIL

Serves 4-6

450 g (1 lb) short pasta (such as penne or rotini)

1 tbsp olive oil

1 cup chopped onion

3 zucchini, halved and sliced

1 cup chopped mushrooms

1 cup sliced celery

1 cup chopped red bell peppers

2 cups cherry tomatoes, halved

2 tbsp olive oil

Green or black olives (optional)

Nutritional yeast (optional)

Pink Himalayan salt

Red pepper chili flakes

1. In large pot of salted boiling water, cook pasta until al dente, about 8 to 9 minutes.

2. In a large skillet, heat oil on medium-high heat. Add onion, zucchini, mushrooms, celery and red peppers. Toss and cook for 5 or 6 minutes. Stir in cherry tomatoes just until warmed.

3. Drain pasta, reserving about 1 cup of pasta water. Return pasta to pot and stir in vegetables. Drizzle olive oil over pasta and toss well.

4. Top with olives, if using. Add pasta water if dry.

5. Stir in nutritional yeast, if using. Season with salt and red pepper chili flakes before serving hot.

SIMPLE SPAGHETTI SAUCE
Serves 4-6

1 tbsp extra-virgin olive or coconut oil

1 onion, diced

2 cloves garlic, minced

1 red bell pepper, diced

1 celery stalk, chopped

1 can (28 oz/796 ml) tomato sauce (with liquid)

1 can (28 oz/796 ml) diced tomatoes (with liquid)

1 can (28 oz/796 ml) whole peeled tomatoes (with liquid)

1 can (5.5 oz/156 ml) tomato paste

1 tbsp dried oregano

Salt and freshly ground black pepper to taste

1. In a medium skillet, heat oil on medium-high heat. Add onion and garlic; cook until onion is softened and translucent.

2. Add red pepper and celery; cook, stirring occasionally, for 5 minutes.

3. Stir in remaining ingredients. Add some water to thin sauce, depending on your preferred thickness.

4. Bring to a boil. Reduce heat; simmer, uncovered, for 3 to 4 hours or until sauce is thickened. The longer you give it time to simmer, the better it tastes.

TIP

- You could add additional vegetables into this sauce, depending on what's in your fridge, including mushrooms, zucchini, carrots or eggplant.

YAM SQUASH SOUP

Serves 4

- 3 baked yams
- 1 spaghetti squash, halved and roasted
- ½ red bell pepper, diced
- 2 cups unsweetened cashew or almond milk (see TIP)
- Salt and freshly ground black pepper
- 2 tbsp curry powder
- 1 tsp turmeric
- 2 green onions, diced
- Handful chopped fresh cilantro
- ¼ cup chopped cashews

1. Remove skin from yams and place flesh in a blender or food processor. Coarsely chop roasted spaghetti squash and add to blender (we use a powerful Vitamix so there's no need for chopping and at times we leave the skin on). Add red pepper to blender.

2. Add enough cashew milk just to cover yams. Blend well for about 1 to 2 minutes. If too thick, add cold water. Stir salt and freshly ground black pepper to taste, along with curry powder and turmeric.

3. Pour yam-squash mixture into a large pot and stir in green onions.

4. Bring pot to stove and cook over medium heat until it begins to boil and warms through.

5. Serve hot in bowls topped with cilantro and a few chopped cashews.

TIP

- You can add more cashew milk for desired consistency just before serving. I also like to add cooked rice to this dish for added texture and flavor.

SWEET POTATO PEANUT STEW

Serves 4

- 1 tsp olive oil or avocado oil
- 1 medium sweet onion, diced
- 2 cloves garlic
- 1 medium sweet potato
- ½ red bell pepper, chopped
- 1 can (28 oz/796 ml) diced tomato (with liquid)
- 4 cups vegetable broth, divided
- ⅓ cup organic peanut butter or almond butter
- 1½ tsp chili powder
- ¼ tsp cayenne powder or to taste
- 1 cup cooked chickpeas
- Handfuls fresh baby spinach
- Sea salt and freshly ground black pepper

1. In a large pot, heat oil on medium-high heat. Sauté onion and garlic until onion is softened and translucent, about 5 minutes.

2. Add sweet potato, red pepper and tomatoes; cook for another 5 minutes.

3. Blend together 1 cup vegetable broth and peanut butter in a blender until mixed. Add mixture to pot with the remaining 3 cups broth, chili powder and cayenne powder. Cover and simmer on medium-low until the sweet potato is tender, about 10 to 20 minutes.

4. Stir in chickpeas and spinach. Season with salt and pepper to taste, and cook until spinach is wilted.

Adapted from The Oh She Glows Cookbook by Angela Liddon

QUINOA SALAD

Serves 2-4

- 1 cup quinoa
- 2 cups water
- 2 tomatoes, diced
- 1 cucumber, diced
- 1 cup chopped fresh parsley
- ½ red onion
- 1 spring onion, sliced
- Olive oil
- Juice of ½ or 1 lemon
- Salt and freshly ground black pepper to taste

1. Rinse quinoa and drain. Place quinoa in a saucepan with the water, bring to a boil, then reduce heat, cover and simmer for 10 minutes until all the water is absorbed. Let it cool completely.

2. Combine cooled quinoa, tomatoes, cucumber, parsley and onions into a large bowl. Toss well. Add olive oil and lemon juice; season with salt and freshly ground black pepper. Toss well and serve.

Adapted from Cooking with Quinoa by Rena Patten

SPICED QUINOA WITH BROCCOLI, ROASTED SWEET POTATO & CRANBERRY SALAD

Serves 2-4

2 medium sweet potatoes, peeled and diced

Olive oil

Salt and freshly ground black pepper to taste

1 cup quinoa, rinsed

½ tsp ground turmeric

1 tsp ground cumin

2 cups water

2 cups broccoli, cut into small florets

⅓ cup dried cranberries

1 green onion, chopped

⅓ cup chopped fresh parsley

Dressing:

1 tbsp olive oil

1 tbsp apple cider vinegar

1½ tbsp balsamic vinegar

Salt and freshly ground black pepper

1. Preheat oven to 400 °F.

2. Place diced sweet potatoes on a large baking sheet drizzled with olive oil and sprinkle with salt and freshly ground black pepper. Roast for 25 to 30 minutes or until golden brown.

3. Combine quinoa, turmeric, cumin and water in a medium saucepan; bring to a boil. Reduce heat to low, cover and simmer for 12 minutes or until water is absorbed. Removed from heat and set aside.

4. Blanch broccoli in a saucepan of boiling water until tender-crisp. Drain and refresh with cold water.

5. For the dressing, whisk together oil, apple cider and balsamic vinegars, salt and freshly ground black pepper.

6. In a large bowl, combine the spiced quinoa, sweet potato, broccoli, cranberries, green onion and parsley.

7. Add dressing to salad and toss well to combine.

Adapted from Supergrains by Chrissy Freer

ZUCCHINI & EGGPLANT SALAD

Serves 4

1 large eggplant

Pinch sea salt

2 tsp avocado oil, divided

4 medium zucchini

1 tsp chili flakes

Freshly ground black pepper to taste

Juice of 1 lemon

1-2 shallots, chopped (or green onion or red onion)

1. Trim and cut unpeeled eggplant lengthwise into 1-inch-thick slices. Sprinkle eggplant slices with salt and let sit for 10 minutes. Rinse eggplant under cool water and pat dry thoroughly.

2. Preheat oven to 400°F. Arrange eggplant in a single layer onto a parchment-lined baking sheet. Sprinkle with half of the oil.

3. Trim and cut zucchini into thin slices. Arrange zucchini in a single layer onto another parchment-lined baking sheet. Sprinkle with remaining oil. Bake both sheet pans for 20 minutes, flipping halfway through cooking, until vegetables are golden-brown and tender.

4. Arrange roasted vegetables on platter and sprinkle with more salt, chili flakes and pepper.

5. Sprinkle with lemon juice and scatter chopped shallots on top.

STUFFED ZUCCHINI
Serves 2-4

2 medium zucchini

1 tbsp avocado oil

½ onion, chopped

1 clove garlic, minced

½ cup chopped mushrooms

½ cup baby spinach

Salt and freshly ground black pepper to taste

Vegan Parmesan cheese (see TIP)

1. Cut zucchini in half lengthwise and remove the pulp from the middle, leaving a ½-inch perimeter.

2. Chop the pulp and set aside.

3. In a medium skillet, heat avocado oil on medium-high heat. Add onion and garlic and cook until onion is softened. Add mushrooms and chopped zucchini. Cook another 5 minutes. Toss in spinach, sprinkle with salt and freshly ground black pepper and cooked for another 1 or 2 minutes until spinach is wilted.

4. Divide the mixture equally and fill zucchini halves with the vegetable mixture. Transfer stuffed zucchini to a greased 9-inch baking pan.

5. Preheat oven 400°F. Bake for 20 minutes or until zucchini are cooked through.

6. Sprinkle tops with vegan Parmesan cheese while hot and serve.

TIP

- See recipe for Vegan Parmesan Cheese on page 166.

EASY GRILLED PEPPERS

Serves 2-4

5 to 6 red bell peppers

1 to 2 tbsp olive oil

1 to 2 tbsp balsamic vinegar

Salt and freshly ground black pepper to taste

1. Trim ends and seed red peppers. Cut into wedges.

2. In a medium bowl, toss pepper wedges with olive oil, vinegar, salt and freshly ground black pepper until well dressed.

3. Preheat oven to 375°F.

4. Place seasoned peppers on a parchment-lined baking sheet.

5. Cook for 45 minutes or until lightly browned. If you prefer them more blistered, cook peppers for 5 more minutes under the broiler.

VARIATION

- You can also grill peppers on the barbeque at medium-high heat. You can either line grill or cookie sheet with aluminum foil to cook peppers.

BRUSCHETTA
Serves 4

4 large tomatoes, chopped

½ cup chopped green onions

1 clove garlic, minced

½ cup minced fresh cilantro

Salt and freshly ground black pepper to taste

4 whole wheat thin hamburger buns or mini pita rounds

Shredded dairy-free cheese

1. In a large bowl, add tomatoes, green onion, garlic and cilantro. Season with salt and pepper. Toss until well combined.

2. Top tomato mixture evenly over whole wheat thin hamburger buns or mini pita rounds.

3. Top with dairy-free cheese.

4. Toast in a preheated barbecue set to medium heat (over indirect heat) until golden brown and cheese is melted. Alternatively, place on baking sheet in a preheated 350°F oven.

GUACAMOLE & NACHOS

Serves 2-4

Guacamole:

3 ripe avocadoes

1 lime

Salt and freshly ground black pepper

½ cup minced red onion (optional)

Hot sauce like Sriracha (optional)

1 cup finely chopped tomatoes

1. Cut 3 ripe avocados lengthwise. Remove pits, but save them! Scoop out avocado into a mixing bowl. Smash with a fork.

2. Cut lime in half and squeeze lime juice from both halves over top avocado. Add salt and freshly ground black pepper to taste. Add onion and hot sauce, if using. Mix well.

3. Stir in tomatoes. Add the pits into the mixture and cover tightly with plastic wrap before storing in refrigerator until ready to serve. The pits prevent the mixture from going brown. Keeps fresh for 1 to 2 days.

Nachos:

1 bag (about 300 or 350 g) whole-grain corn tortilla chips

1 jar (14 oz/418 ml) salsa

2 cups shredded dairy-free cheese, divided

Black olives

Chopped tomatoes

Chopped red bell peppers

Sliced green onions

Freshly chopped lettuce or cilantro (optional)

1. Preheat oven to 350°F. On a baking sheet, spread tortilla chips in a single layer.

2. Spread salsa on chips, followed by a layer of cheese.

3. Sprinkle a handful each of black olives, tomatoes, red peppers and green onions, if using.

4. Bake in oven for 30 minutes. Set oven to broil and cook for another 5 minutes until cheese is golden.

5. Remove from oven and cover with freshly chopped lettuce or cilantro, if using.

SPAGHETTI SQUASH

Serves 2-4

1 spaghetti squash

Olive, coconut or avocado oil

Salt and freshly ground black pepper

1. Preheat oven to 400°F. Line a large, rimmed baking sheet with parchment paper.

2. Cut spaghetti squash in half. Use a large spoon to scoop out seeds and discard them.

3. Drizzle the insides of each squash half with 1 tsp olive oil and rub it all over the inside, adding more oil if necessary. Sprinkle with salt and freshly ground black pepper lightly over the squash.

4. Place both halves cut-side down on prepared baking sheet.

5. Bake for 40 to 60 minutes, until the cut sides are turning golden and they are easily pierced with a fork. (Smaller squash will cook sooner.)

6. Once the squash is done baking, use a fork to fluff the insides to resemble spaghetti. Serve as is or topped with desired sauce.

STUFFED MUSHROOMS
Serves 5-6

20 small or 10 medium cremini mushrooms

1 tsp extra-virgin olive oil or avocado oil

¼ cup raw almonds

½ medium onion, roughly chopped

1½ tbsp organic tamari

1 tbsp balsamic vinegar

2 cloves garlic, chopped

1 tbsp chopped fresh rosemary or 1 tsp dried rosemary

1. Preheat oven to 350°F.

2. Wipe mushrooms with kitchen paper or clean cloth. Gently remove stems.

3. Grease an 8 x 8-inch baking pan with olive oil, then place mushroom caps in dish with stemless side up.

4. In a food processor, pulse almonds until fine; add remaining ingredients and continue to process until smooth. Fill mushrooms evenly with mixture. Scatter mushroom stems in between caps.

5. Bake for 30 minutes or until filling is golden.

Excerpted from Alive Calendar Cookbook

VEGAN PARMESAN CHEESE

Makes 1 cup

1 cup raw cashew or walnuts
4 tbsp nutritional yeast
1 tsp garlic powder
1 tsp salt

1. Add all ingredients to a food processor and blend until well mixed.

2. Store in a glass jar. Keep refrigerated—it keeps well for several weeks.

TIP

- This versatile "cheese" topping goes well when sprinkled on any veggie. Try it on the Stuffed Zucchini recipe on page 159.

Adapted from simpleveganblog.com

VEGAN SOUR CREAM

Makes 2 cups

- 1½ **cups raw cashews**
- **1 cup water, or as needed**
- **2 tbsp freshly squeezed lemon juice**
- ½ **tsp salt to taste**
- ¼ **tsp nutritional yeast**

1. Soak cashews overnight or in boiling water for 30 to 60 minutes. Drain and rinse.

2. In a food processor, add cashews, water, lemon juice, salt and nutritional yeast. Process until smooth, scraping down the sides of food processor, if necessary.

3. Transfer cream to an airtight container and refrigerate until ready to use. The sour cream will stay fresh in the fridge for 1 week or in the freezer for about 4 weeks.

TIP

- This sour cream tastes great on a baked potato or sweet potato, nachos or Tex-Mex wrap.

CHOCO-NUT ENERGY BALLS

Makes 10-15 energy balls

¾ cup pitted dates

1 cup raw walnuts or almonds

⅓ cup cacao nibs

3 tbsp raw cacao powder

4 tbsp hemp seeds, divided

1 tsp vanilla extract

Pinch sea salt

1 cup unsweetened organic shredded coconut

1. In a medium bowl, soak dates in lukewarm water for 30 minutes. Drain and set aside.

2. In a food processor, pulse walnuts until they resemble coarse crumbs.

3. Add soaked dates, cacao nibs, cacao powder, 2 tablespoons hemp seeds, vanilla and salt to processor. Pulse until well incorporated and forms a "dough" ball.

4. In a shallow bowl, add shredded coconut and remaining hemp seeds. Toss to combine.

5. Roll 2 tablespoons of the dough at a time between your hands to form small balls. (Use a tiny amount of oil on the palms of your hands if they get sticky.)

6. Place energy balls in coconut-hemp seeds mixture. Roll until covered.

TIP

- These energy balls are delicious any time of the day when hunger strikes and can be stored in an airtight container in the fridge for up to a week.

CHOCOLATE ALMOND BUTTER FUDGE

Makes 15 to 20 pieces

2 cups almond butter or natural peanut butter

¼ cup raw cacao powder

½ cup maple syrup

1 tsp coconut oil

1 tbsp vanilla extract

1 tsp sea salt

1. In a large bowl, combine all ingredients and stir well. Scrape the mixture into a square 8 x 8-inch baking pan, lined with parchment paper. Flatten mixture well with a spatula.

2. Freeze and chill for 1 to 2 hours. Remove fudge from freezer and cut into small squares.

3. Store in an airtight container or resealable freezer bag; place back in freezer to keep cool before serving.

VEGAN CHOCOLATE CAKE

Makes about 12 slices, one 8-inch cake

Cake:

1½ cups + 2 tbsp all-purpose flour

1½ tsp baking soda

½ tsp sea salt

1½ tsp instant coffee

¾ cup unsweetened cocoa powder

1 cup + 3 tbsp dark brown sugar

1½ cups hot water

¾ cup + 2 tbsp coconut oil

1½ tsp apple cider vinegar

Icing:

¼ cup + 1 tbsp coconut butter (not the same as oil)

¼ cup dark brown sugar

1½ tsp instant coffee

1½ tbsp cocoa powder

¾ cup finely chopped dark baking chocolate (at least
    70% cocoa)

Garnish:

1 tbsp pistachios, chopped

Cake:

1. Preheat oven to 350°F.

2. Spray the sides of an 8 x 8-inch square baking pan or round cake pan with cooking spray, then line the bottom of pan with parchment paper.

3. In a large bowl, combine flour, baking soda, salt, instant coffee and cocoa powder; stir until well combined.

4. In a second bowl, mix together sugar, hot water, coconut oil and apple cider vinegar until coconut oil has dissolved. Stir into the dry ingredients.

5. Pour batter into prepared baking pan and bake until a pick inserted in the center comes out clean, about 35 minutes. (You know it's ready when the cake is coming away from the edges of the pan slightly.)

6. Transfer pan to a wire rack and let cake cool in pan. Once cooled, remove from pan to a serving dish.

Icing:

1. For the icing, add all icing ingredients, except for chopped chocolate, into a heavy-based saucepan and add 4 tablespoons cold water. Bring to a boil. Once everything is dissolved, turn off heat.

2. Add chopped chocolate and swirl the pan so that the chocolate is all covered and allow it to sit for 1 minute. Whisk until you have a dark glossy icing, and leave to cool until runny enough to cover the cake, but thick enough to stay mostly on top.

3. Pour icing over cake, using a spatula to ease the icing to the edges.

4. Decorate with chopped pistachios while the icing is still slightly warm.

5. Leave to stand for 30 minutes for the icing to set before slicing the cake.

Excerpted from Goodness Me Natural Food Market magazine

The Wheels of Health Daily Log

"YOU GET WHAT YOU MEASURE"

There's an old saying—unless you measure it, it won't happen. I have made it a habit over the last 10 years of tracking my eating, exercise, sleep and mindful practices. I keep my log on my night table and take a few minutes every night to summarize my day before going to bed. On days where I do great and give myself "good marks," it feels so good. On days when things don't go as planned, it allows me to reflect on the reasons I didn't reach my targets and make plans to get on track the next day.

I suggest you print off a week's worth of copies and complete this log every day for an entire week. If you're like me, you'll be hooked and it will make a big difference in helping to balance your Wheels of Health and keep you on target by charting small gains. Over time, charting your progress will encourage you to always do better next time.

Page 173 is a completed copy as an example, while page 174 is a blank version for you to copy and fill out.

You can also access an electronic copy and complete it online if you wish by going to advicahealth.com/nevertoolatetobehealthy/.

The Wheels of Health Daily Log   DATE: 3/12/21

EATING WELL

SUPPLEMENTS: Probiotics, Vitamin D, multivitamin

BREAKFAST: Shake (spinach, blueberries, protein)

LUNCH: Large salad, rice, sweet potato

DINNER: Quinoa burger (2), salad

SNACKS: Almond butter fudge   ALCOHOL: None

EXERCISE

ACTIVITY: Cycling   INTENSITY: Hard

TIME: 2 hrs 15 minutes   DISTANCE: 58 km

DESCRIPTION: Did Rosseau Loop, went hard, felt good

SLEEP

HOURS: 7.5 hours   QUALITY: Good

MINDFULNESS

STRESS REDUCTION: Deep-breathing exercises

REFLECTION

HOW DID YOU DO?

(AMAZING)   SATISFACTORY   UNSATISFACTORY

GOALS FOR TOMORROW: Cut down coffee to 2 cups,

8 hours sleep

The Wheels of Health Daily Log   DATE: /   /

EATING WELL

SUPPLEMENTS:_____

BREAKFAST:_____

LUNCH: _____

DINNER: _____

SNACKS: _____   ALCOHOL: _____

EXERCISE

ACTIVITY:_____   INTENSITY:_____

TIME:_____   DISTANCE: _____

DESCRIPTION: _____

_____

_____

SLEEP

HOURS: _____   QUALITY: _____

MINDFULNESS

STRESS REDUCTION: _____

REFLECTION

HOW DID YOU DO?

AMAZING   SATISFACTORY   UNSATISFACTORY

GOALS FOR TOMORROW: _____

_____

_____

_____

Kevin's Top Picks

TOP BOOKS

Each of the books I list below have had a significant effect on my life and my family's. In fact, I've read many of the books below several times and use them as ongoing resources to continually improve my health. I make a habit of reading every night before I go to sleep.

Boundless by Ben Greenfield

Chris Beat Cancer by Chris Work

Engine 2 Diet by Rip Esselstyn

Finding Ultra by Rich Roll

How Not To Die by Michael Greger

Radical Remission by Kelly Turner

Superlife by Darin Olien

The Blue Zones by Dan Buettner

The China Study by Colin C. Campbell

Own the Day by Aubrey Markus

TOP PODCASTS

I love listening to podcasts while I'm driving or during my downtime. Here are some of my favorites—in fact, I often find it tough to decide which one I listen to first since they're all amazing shows.

For the Life of Me, hosted by Julie Piatt

Impact Theory, hosted by Tom Bilyeu

Living Beyond 120, hosted by Dr. Jeff Gladden and Dr. Mark Young

NutritionFacts.com, hosted by Michael Greger

On Purpose, hosted by Jay Shetty

Optimize, hosted by Brian Johnson

Plant Strong, hosted by Rip Esselstyn

The Ben Greenfield Podcast

The Darin Olien Show

The Rich Roll Podcast, hosted by Rich Roll

TOP HEALTH MOVIES/DOCUMENTARIES

These movies have had a dramatic effect on my health and my life. They've also taught me so much about the health benefits of eating a plant-based diet. I've watched some of these movies at least three times.

Down To Earth (2020)

The Game Changers (2019)

What the Health (2017)

Cowspiracy (2014)

Forks Over Knives (2011)

Fat, Sick & Nearly Dead (2010)

References

Page 5
Greger, M., & Stone, G. (2015). *How not to die: Discover the foods scientifically proven to prevent and reverse disease*. Flatiron Books.

Research and Markets. (2019). *The U.S weight loss and diet control market*. https://www.researchandmarkets.com/research/6sb283/united_states?w=5

Page 6
Wennberg, A. M., Wu, M. N., Rosenberg, P. B., & Spira, A. P. (2017, August). Sleep disturbance, cognitive decline, and dementia: a review. In *Seminars in neurology* (Vol. 37, No. 4, p. 395).

Page 10
Centres for Disease Control (CDC). (n.d.). *Heart disease and stroke prevention: time for action*. [PDF file]. https://www.cdc.gov/dhdsp/action_plan/pdfs/action_plan_30f7.pdf

Public Health Ontario. (2019). *The burden of chronic diseases in Canada: key estimates to support efforts in prevention*. https://www.publichealthontario.ca/-/media/documents/c/2019/cdburden-report.pdf?la=en

Harvard T.H. Chan School of Public Health. (2020). *The nutrition source: diabetes*. https://www.hsph.harvard.edu/nutritionsource/disease-prevention/diabetes-prevention/

Page 13
Keating, L. (2017). *Survey finds most people check their smartphones before getting out of bed in the morning*. Tech Times. https://www.techtimes.com/articles/199967/20170302/survey-finds-people-check-smartphones-before-getting-out-bed.htm

Page 19
Hew-Butler, T., Loi, V., Pani, A., & Rosner, M. H. (2017). Exercise-associated hyponatremia: 2017 update. *Frontiers in medicine*, 4, 21.

Siegel, A. J., Verbalis, J. G., Clement, S., Mendelson, J. H., Mello, N. K., Adner, M., ... & Lewandrowski, K. B. (2007). Hyponatremia in marathon runners due to inappropriate arginine vasopressin secretion. *The American journal of medicine*, 120(5), 461-e11.

Page 30
Hyman, M. Dairy: 6 Reasons You Should Avoid it at All Costs or Why Following the USDA Food Pyramid Guidelines is Bad for Your Health. *health*, 416, 884-5911.

Page 34
Jacques, R. (2017). *These disturbing fast food truths will make you reconsider your lunch*. Huffington Post. https://www.huffingtonpost.ca/entry/fast-food-truths_n_4296243

Page 42
Goldhamer, A. (2020). *Your body heals itself*. Colin Campbell Centre for Nutrition Studies. https://nutritionstudies.org/body-heals/

Page 46
Moubarac, J.C. (2017). *Ultra-processed foods in Canada: consumption, impact on diet quality and policy implications*. Heart and Stroke Foundation Canada. https://www.heartandstroke.ca/-/media/pdf-files/canada/media-centre/hs-report-upp-moubarac-dec-5-2017.ashx

Standard American diet. (n.d.). Nutrition Facts.org. https://nutritionfacts.org/topics/standard-american-diet/

Dupont Nutrition & Biosciences. (2018). *Plant-based eating: Nearly seven of 10 Americans trying to increase plant protein consumption*. Food Navigator USA. *https://www.foodnavigator-usa.com/News/Promotional-Features/MEGATREND-Plant-based-eating-Nearly-seven-of-10-*

Americans-trying-to-increase-plant-protein-consumption

Buzby, J.C. (2008). *Dietary assessment of major trends in U.S. food consumption, 1970-2005*. United States Department of Agriculture. https://www.ers.usda.gov/

Page 47
Kim, H., Caulfield, L. E., Garcia-Larsen, V., Steffen, L. M., Coresh, J., & Rebholz, C. M. (2019). Plant-Based diets are associated with a lower risk of incident cardiovascular disease, cardiovascular disease mortality, and All-Cause mortality in a general population of Middle-Aged adults. *Journal of the American Heart Association*, 8(16).

Page 48/49
Buettner, D. (2015). *The blue zone's solution: Eating and living like the world's healthiest people.* (1st ed.). National Geographic.

Greger, M., & Stone, G. (2015). *How not to die: Discover the foods scientifically proven to prevent and reverse disease.* Flatiron Books.

Page 50
DYLN Inc. (2014). *8 reasons to start your day with lemon water*. Mind & Body. https://www.dyln.co/blogs/y-blog/18464135-8-reasons-to-start-your-day-with-lemon-water

Johnston, C. S., & Gaas, C. A. (2006). Vinegar: medicinal uses and antiglycemic effect. *Medscape General Medicine*, 8(2), 61.

Gunnars, K. (2020). *6 health benefits of apple cider vinegar, backed by science.* Healthline. https://www.healthline.com/nutrition/6-proven-health-benefits-of-apple-cider-vinegar

Khezri, S. S., Saidpour, A., Hosseinzadeh, N., & Amiri, Z. (2018). Beneficial effects of apple cider vinegar on weight management, Visceral Adiposity Index and lipid profile in overweight or obese subjects receiving restricted calorie diet: A randomized clinical trial. *Journal of functional foods*, 43, 95-102.

Berry, J. (2018). *Health benefits of apple cider vinegar.* Medical News Today. https://www.medicalnewstoday.com/articles/323721

Page 51
Hendricks, S. (2017). *It turns out you can drink too much apple cider vinegar: Here's what you should know.* Insider. https://www.insider.com/can-you-drink-too-much-apple-cider-vinegar-2019-2#:~:text=But%20too%20much%20apple%20cider,diluted%20and%20with%20other%20food.

He, Y., Yue Y., Zheng X., Zhang K., Chen S., & Du Z. (2015). Curcumin, inflammation, and chronic diseases: how are they linked? *Molecules*, 20(5):9183-213.

Jurenka, J.S. (2009). Anti-inflammatory properties of curcumin, a major constituent of Curcuma longa: a review of preclinical and clinical research. *Altern Med Rev*, 14(2):141-53.

Mann, T. (2018). *Why do dieters regain weight?.* American Psychological Association. https://www.apa.org/science/about/psa/2018/05/calorie-deprivation

Page 55
David Suzuki Foundation. (2020). *Food and climate change.* https://davidsuzuki.org/queen-of-green/food-climate-change/

Campbell, T. C., & Campbell, T. M. (2005). *The China study: The most comprehensive study of nutrition ever conducted and the startling implications for diet, weight loss and long-term health.* BenBella Books.

Longo, V. (2018). *The longevity diet: discover the new science behind stem cell activation and regeneration to slow aging, fight disease, and optimize weight.* Avery.

Page 59
Buettner, D. (2015). *The blue zone's solution: Eating and living like the world's healthiest people.* (1st ed.). National Geographic.

Page 60

Watson, K. (2017). *Cold shower benefits for your health.* Healthline. https://www.healthline.com/health/cold-shower-benefits

Page 61

Siems, W. G., van Kuijk, F. J., Maass, R., & Brenke, R. (1994). Uric acid and glutathione levels during short-term whole body cold exposure. *Free Radical Biology and Medicine,* 16(3), 299-305.

Siems, W. G., van Kuijk, F. J., Maass, R., & Brenke, R. (1994). Uric acid and glutathione levels during short-term whole body cold exposure. *Free Radical Biology and Medicine,* 16(3), 299-305.

Page 62

The Mayo Clinic. (2020). *Exercise and stress: Get moving to manage stress.* https://www.mayoclinic.org/healthy-lifestyle/stress-management/in-depth/exercise-and-stress/art-20044469#:~:text=-Regular%20exercise%20can%20increase%20self,by%20stress%2C%20depression%20and%20anxiety.

Page 63

Harvard Health Publishing. (2010). *A prescription for better health: go alfresco.* https://www.health.harvard.edu/newsletter_article/a-prescription-for-better-health-go-alfresco

Wilson, E. O. (2017). Biophilia and the conservation ethic. In D.J Penn, & I. Mysterud (Eds), *Evolutionary perspectives on environmental problems* (pp. 263-272). Routledge.

Mark, J. (2018). Get Out of Here: Scientists Examine the Benefits of Forests, Birdsong and Running Water. The New York Times. https://www.nytimes.com/2017/03/02/books/review/nature-fix-florence-williams.html

Weir, K. (2020). *Nurtured by nature.* https://www.apa.org/monitor/2020/04/nurtured-nature

Sarkar, A., Lehto, S. M., Harty, S., Dinan, T. G., Cryan, J. F., & Burnet, P. W. (2016). Psychobiotics and the manipulation of bacteria–gut–brain signals. *Trends in neurosciences,* 39(11), 763-781.

Page 64

Alzheimers Society. (n.d.). How to reduce your risk of dementia. https://www.alzheimers.org.uk/about-dementia/risk-factors-and-prevention/how-reduce-your-risk-dementia

Page 66

Government of Canada. (2019). *Are Canadians getting enough sleep?* Public Health Agency of Canada. https://www.canada.ca/en/public-health/services/publications/healthy-living/canadian-adults-get-ting-enough-sleep-info-graphic.html

Centre for Disease Control and Prevention. (2017). *Sleep and sleep disorders.* https://www.cdc.gov/sleep/data_statistics.html

Page 67

Harvard Medical. Why do we sleep, anyway? Healthy Sleep. http://healthysleep.med.harvard.edu/healthy/matters/benefits-of-sleep/why-do-we-sleep

Leech, J. (2020). *10 reasons why good sleep is important.* Healthline. https://www.healthline.com/nutrition/10-reasons-why-good-sleep-is-important

National Institute of Health. (2020). *Magnesium: fact sheet for health professionals.* Office of Dietary Supplements. https://ods.od.nih.gov/factsheets/Magnesium-HealthProfessional/#:~:text=Magnesium%20is%20widely%20distributed%20in,cereals%20and%20other%20fortified%20foods.

Breus, M. (2019). *3 Amazing benefits of GABA.* Psychology Today. https://www.psychologytoday.com/ca/blog/sleep-newzzz/201901/3-amazing-benefits-gaba

Kim, S., Jo, K., Hong, K. B., Han, S. H., & Suh, H. J. (2019). GABA and l-theanine mixture decreases sleep latency and improves

NREM sleep. *Pharmaceutical biology*, 57(1), 64-72.

Page 68
National Institute of Health. (2019). *What does zinc do?* Office of Dietary Supplements. https://ods.od.nih.gov/factsheets/Zinc-Consumer/

Page 70
Harper, K. (2015). *The science of sleep*. American Chemical Society. https://www.acs.org/content/acs/en/education/resources/highschool/chemmatters/past-issues/archive-2014-2015/the-science-of-sleep.html

Sleep Foundation.org. (2020). *What your sleep habits reveal about your dementia risk*. Sleep Topics. https://www.sleepfoundation.org/articles/what-your-sleep-habits-reveal-about-your-dementia-risk

National Institute of Health. (2018). *Sleep deprivation increases Alzheimer's protein*. NIH Research Matters. https://www.nih.gov/news-events/nih-research-matters/sleep-deprivation-increases-alzheimers-protein

Sleep Foundation.org. (2020). *Parkinson's disease and sleep*. Sleep Topics. https://www.sleepfoundation.org/articles/parkinsons-disease-and-sleep

National Institute of Health. (2013). *Brain may flush out toxins during sleep:* NIH-*funded study suggests sleep clears brain of damaging molecules associated with neurodegeneration*. News Releases. https://www.nih.gov/news-events/news-releases/brain-may-flush-out-toxins-during-sleep

Page 71
Winter, M.C. (2017). *The Sleep Solution: Why your sleep is broken and how to fix it*. Berkley.

Page 73
Zaccaro, A., Piarulli, A., Laurino, M., Garbella, E., Menicucci, D., Neri, B., & Gemignani, A. (2018). How breath-control can change your life: a systematic review on psycho-physiological correlates of slow breathing. *Frontiers in human neuroscience*, 12, 353.

Brown, R., & Gerbarg, P. (2012). *The healing power of the breath: Simple techniques to reduce stress and anxiety, enhance concentration, and balance your emotions*. Shambhala Publications, 2012.

Page 76
Morin, M. (2017). *13 things mentally strong people do: Take Back Your Power, Embrace Change, Face Your Fears, and Train Your Brain for Happiness and Success*. William Morrow Paperbacks.

Morin, A. (2015). 7 Scientifically Proven Benefits of Gratitude/ Psychology Today. https://www.psychologytoday.com/ca/blog/what-mentally-strong-people-dont-do/201504/7-scientifically-proven-benefits-gratitude

Page 77
Wood, A. M., Joseph, S., Lloyd, J., & Atkins, S. (2009). Gratitude influences sleep through the mechanism of pre-sleep cognitions. Journal of psychosomatic research, 66(1), 43-48.

Wong, Y. J., Owen, J., Gabana, N. T., Brown, J. W., McInnis, S., Toth, P., & Gilman, L. (2018). Does gratitude writing improve the mental health of psychotherapy clients? Evidence from a randomized controlled trial. *Psychotherapy Research*, 28(2), 192-202.

Page 79
Barrett, C. J. (2017). Mindfulness and rehabilitation: Teaching yoga and meditation to young men in an alternative to incarceration program. International journal of offender therapy and comparative criminology, 61(15), 1719-1738.

Mayo Clinic. (2020). Meditation: A simple, fast way to reduce stress. https://www.mayoclinic.org/tests-procedures/meditation/in-depth/meditation/art-20045858

Page 82
Borresen, K. (2020). The psychological benefits of having things to look

forward to. Huffington Post. https://www.huffingtonpost.ca/entry/psychological-benefits-things-look-forward-to_l_5ec40575c5b-62696fb60e3a1

Kumar, A., Killingsworth, M. A., & Gilovich, T. (2014). Waiting for merlot: Anticipatory consumption of experiential and material purchases. Psychological science, 25(10), 1924-1931.

Niven, D. (2000). The 100 simple secrets of happy people. Harper San Francisco.

Page 83
Burzynska, B. (2018). Gratitude contemplation as a method to improve human well-being and physical functioning: theoretical review of existing research. *Journal of Education, Health and Sport, 8*(3), 298-311.

Harvard Health Publishing. (n.d.). *7 ways to keep your memory sharp at any age*. Healthbeat. https://www.health.harvard.edu/healthbeat/7-ways-to-keep-your-memory-sharp-at-any-age

Park, D. C., Lodi-Smith, J., Drew, L., Haber, S., Hebrank, A., Bischof, G. N., & Aamodt, W. (2014). The impact of sustained engagement on cognitive function in older adults: the synapse project. *Psychological science, 25*(1), 103-112.

National Institute on Aging. (2020). *Cognitive health and older adults.* Cognitive Health. https://www.nia.nih.gov/health/cognitive-health-and-older-adults

Page 84
The Tim Ferriss Show. (2015). The magic of mindfulness: Complain less, appreciate more, and live a better life (#122). https://tim.blog/2015/11/29/magic-of-mindfulness/

Page 96
Hoffman, J. (2012). *The anxiety of waiting for test results.* The New York Times. https://well.blogs.nytimes.com/2012/07/23/the-anxiety-of-waiting-for-test-results/

Page 99
Turner, N. (1997). *The Hormone Diet: A 3-Step Program to Help You Lose Weight, Gain Strength, and Live Younger Longer.* Rodale Books.

Page 108
Andersen, J. (2020). *Marathon statistics 2019 worldwide.* https://runrepeat.com/research-marathon-performance-across-nations

Gough, C. (2018). *Running and jogging: Statistics and facts.* https://www.statista.com/topics/1743/running-and-jogging/

Gough, C. (2020). *Total number of memberships at fitness centres/ health clubs*

in the U.S. from 2000 to 2017. Statistics. https://www.statista.com/statistics/236123/us-fitness-center--health-club-memberships/

Hoffman, K. (2020). *41 New Fitness & Gym Membership Statistics for 2020.* Noob Gains. https://noobgains.com/gym-membership-statistics/

Lange, D. (2019). *Fitness industry in Europe: Statistics & facts.* Statistica. https://www.statista.com/topics/3405/fitness-industry-in-europe/

Page 110
O'Brien, E. (2003). Employers' benefits from workers' health insurance. *The Milbank Quarterly, 81*(1), 5-43.

Sun Life Financial. (2016). *Sun Life—Ivey Canadian wellness ROI study update.* https://www.sunlife.ca/static/canada/Sponsor/About%20Group%20Benefits/Group%20benefits%20products%20and%20services/Health%20and%20wellness/Wellness%20ROI%20Study/Files/PDF7224-E.pdf

Page 111
Gubler, T., Larkin, I., & Pierce, L. (2018). Doing well by making well: The impact of corporate wellness programs on employee productivity. *Management Science, 64*(11), 4967-4987.

Page 113

Rochon, P.A., Schmader, K., & Givens, J. (2020). *Drug prescribing in older adults.* https://www.uptodate.com/contents/drug-prescribing-for-older-adults

Dagli, R. J., & Sharma, A. (2014). Polypharmacy: a global risk factor for elderly people. *Journal of international oral health: JIOH, 6(6).*

Harvard Health Publishing. (2016). *7 things you can do to avoid drug interactions.* https://www.health.harvard.edu/staying-healthy/7-things-you-can-do-to-avoid-drug-interactions

Recipe Resource List

America's Test Kitchen. (2017). *Vegan for Everybody: Foolproof plant-based recipes for breakfast, lunch, dinner and in between.* America's Test Kitchen.

Fetterly, N. (2015). *Almond tamari stuffed mushrooms.* Alive.com. https://www.alive.com/recipe/almond-tamari-stuffed-mushrooms/

Freer, C. (2013). *Supergrains: Cook your way to great health.* Appetite by Random House.

Green, P. (2011). *Quinoa 365: The everyday superfood.* Whitecap Books.

Liddon, A. (2014). *The Oh She Glows Cookbook: Vegan recipes to glow from the inside out.* Penguin Canada.

Patten, R. (2011). *Cooking with Quinoa: The supergrain.* New Holland Publishers.

Romero, T.H. (2016). *Protein Ninja: Power through your day with 100 hearty plant-based recipes that pack a protein punch.* Da Capo Lifelong Books.

Vegan parmesan cheese. (2020). Simple Vegan Blog. https://simpleveganblog.com/vegan-parmesan-cheese/

To learn more about Kevin's journey to peak health, stay connected

ADVICA HEALTH

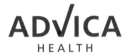

Health Blog & Podcasts: advicahealth.com/blog/

Instagram: @advica.health

Linkedin: linkedin.com/company/advicahealth

Twitter: @advicahealth

KEVIN BRADY

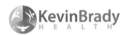

Health blog: kevinbradyhealth.ca/

Instagram: @kevinbradyhealth

Linkedin: linkedin.com/in/kevin-brady-32a363110/

Podcasts: kevinbradyhealth.ca/podcasts/

OTHER PUBLICATIONS BY KEVIN BRADY

Return on Wellness e-book: advicahealth.com/corporate/

MORE PRAISE FOR
It's Never Too Late to Be Healthy

"What impressed me most as I read Kevin's book was his commitment to family. Families are the building blocks of a healthy society. Health starts at home. It is impressive to get a glimpse of what a high-functioning family looks like. Thanks for sharing Kev." –Mary Maciel Pearson, health and wellness consultant

"Kevin inspires me every day to make health, fitness and longevity my No. 1 priority, and his book provides a game-changing roadmap for all CEOs to take action now!" –Nancy MacKay, CEO and Founder, MacKay CEO Forums

"Kevin brings a lifetime of personal experience from his own journey to his book. His deep commitment to his health and that of his clients has taken him on a journey of learning from some of the best in the field. This is a must read for those who want to raise the bar on their own health and wellness." –Bruce Bowser, chair of the board at AMJ Campbell Van Lines and author of *The Focus Effect: Change Your Work, Change Your Life*

"Finally! *It's Never Too Late To Be Healthy* releases you from the burden of weeding through the vast amount of health and wellness information out there. Kevin's book is relatable, vulnerable, comprehensive and enjoyable to read. I'm sharing it with every client and student across the planet!" –Nicolette Richer, MA, PhD candidate, CEO & Founder, Green Moustache Juice Inc & Richer Health Consulting Inc.

"Kev's advice is ridiculously balanced and useful. His health practices for the most part aren't about restriction (hey, Kevin himself eats fudge nearly every night). His practices are more about little additions to your daily routine that produce noticeable results. If you're in your 30s, 40s, 50s, 60s, or 70s, boy, are you in for a productive read that'll have implications in every part of your life." –Mark Levy, Founder and CEO, Levy Innovation: A Strategy and Differentiation Company